"Chemical Free Pets"

Nancy Brandt DVM, CVC, CVA

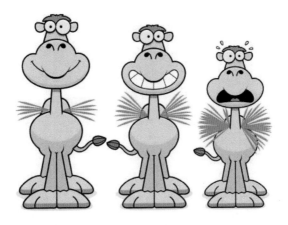

Ordering Information:
www.safe4animals.com

www.safearomatherapy.com

Printed in the United States of America

Dedication

For all my Furry Friends that taught me all about medicine and love.

To all our furry pets that are joining us in holding this Earth sacred.

Thank you to all of my readers who are endeavoring to bless all inhabitants of this planet.

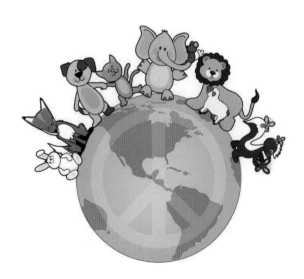

Congratulations!!

In my practice I tell everyone that I have the Best of the Best clients ever and it is true!! Why you ask – because any animal guardian who commits to a holistic life style does so because they value the life of their pet highly. That's the Best. The reason I do what I do is to preserve the relationship we forge with our furry ones as long as possible.

You are the Best!! That's you for picking up this book. Your commitment to your whole family those furry ones included, is to be commended.

A "Wholistic" life is investigating the whole aspect of impact on our biological systems. This book educates you, the guardian; on the many areas chemicals impact your pet's health. I then give fabulous alternatives that decrease the toxic load or burden our pets are forced to carry. It all adds up.

Introduction

This book developed out of a need to assist my clients in "Cleaning House". I wanted to supply a check list of What, Where and How to discover hidden dangers. Those "Straws on the Camel's Back" that go uncounted often.

Not any one toxin, chemical or artificial substance will be the item to sacrifice your pets' life. It takes them all adding up to become a burden to a biological system and cause DIS-EASE. The more areas we control the less taxed your pet's biological system will be. The less straws over time on the camel's back the longer they are with us to love and cuddle.

Over 20 years of introducing healthy alternatives this book shares with you the Best of the Best for your pets.

Be a Blessed

Blessing Always,

Dr. Nancy

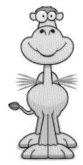

Disclaimer:

The information presented herein is in no way intended to treat, cure, diagnose or prevent any disease or illness. If you feel you have a medical condition you are urged to seek the help of a medical professional. You are encouraged to first seek the counsel of your health care professional before making any changes to your current health routine. The suggestions in this book are for use with Therapeutic Grade Essential Oils as appropriately labeled for use. This book is being distributed with the understanding that the publisher and the authors are not liable for the misconception or misuse of the information provided.

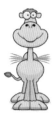

TABLE OF CONTENTS

CHAPTER ONE: Chemical Dangers

Too many straws on the camel's back adds up to
TOXIC. Toxic is a state of ………

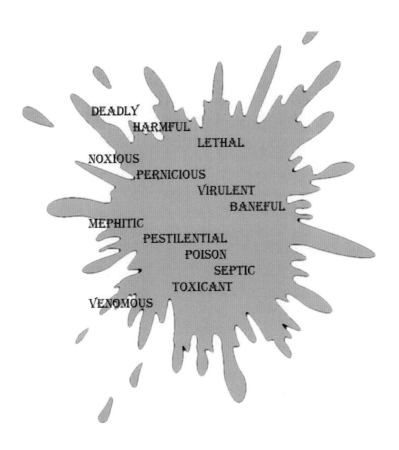

DEADLY
HARMFUL
LETHAL
NOXIOUS
PERNICIOUS
VIRULENT
BANEFUL
MEPHITIC
PESTILENTIAL
POISON
SEPTIC
TOXICANT
VENOMOUS

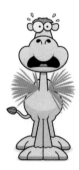

A Biological System in DIS-EASE or DIS-FUNCTION!!!!

The **Toxic Substance Control Act (TSCA)** of 1976 grandfathered in estimated 65,000-100,000 chemicals currently on the market today. What does this mean to you? It simply means – "These chemicals have not had any safety testing and we know very little information about their effects." Of the chemicals tested, toxic labeling is required only if 50% or more of the animals tested with a chemical die. Under the TSCA, manufacturers are protected by trade secret laws that allow them to keep their ingredient lists a secret. "It is unthinkable that anyone would knowingly inflict such exposures on their families, pets and themselves, if products routinely used were labeled with explicit warning of cancer risks' " says Dr. Samuel Epstein, chairman of the Cancer Prevention Coalition and emeritus Professor of Occupational and Environmental Medicine at the University of Illinois, School of Public Health at Chicago, and leading international authority on 'toxicology' and the carcinogenic effects of contaminants in consumer products.

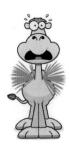

The rise in disease has many factors; there is an aging population, an increase in obesity and a significant increase in the toxicity of the world. Our pets are also falling prey to age, obesity and toxicity.

What we think to be safe and often choose with the best of intents frequently is self-intoxicating. Even with exhaustive Google research we fall prey to the extensive marketing ploys of the consumer goods driven economy. Safety tests are often done on a group of animals that are healthy and young. Many studies are deemed safe if only 50% of the animals die in the study. So they are saying a 50:50 chance of being safe as long as the biological system is healthy and young. That is not safe for me. If an airline had a 50% safety rating I would not fly them.

"The American Cancer Society estimates a 50% rise in cancer rates by the year 2020."

To follow are checklists of where to look, what to look for and how to create alternatives. In the end we do all that we can do and that is always enough; when we do all we can do because we love and cherish those family members with the wiggly tails that is always enough. Use this book to create awareness and alternatives to make the planet safer for us all to continue to inhabit for millions of years to come.

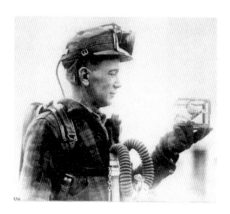

Pet's as Sentinels

There are toxic chemicals found in our pets at alarming levels according to a study in Virginia by the Environmental Working Group (EWG); overall 35 chemicals in dogs and 46 chemicals in cats were found. For example:

Brominated flame retardants in cats were 23X higher than in humans

Mercury levels in cats were 5X higher

Perifluorinated chemicals were 2.4X higher in dogs

"We need a better system of regulating toxic chemicals in this country," said Bill Walker, vice president of the west coast Environmental Working Group, "We need to test the chemicals before they are allowed on the market. Our animals are trying to tell us something here."

With the impact of our environment upon us and us upon it, now is the time to notice the effects of our choices. Animals are upwards of 40 times more affected by the pollution in the environment. It stands to reason that if we are to impact the environment in a positive manner we must do so with natural products not those synthetically created in a laboratory. Essential Oils are a logical choice. Veterinary Medical Aromatherapy ® plays a role now in the health and well-being of our pets.

The National Research Council has found that sickness and disease in pets can inform our understanding of our own health risks. (NRC 1991) Similar studies have been conducted in people by the Centers of Disease Control and Prevention (CDC) and EWG and found that animals show significantly higher amounts of the chemicals known to cause disease in people. For example:

Teflon   2.4X higher in dogs

Why is this significant? As we see an increase in disease in animals so shall we see an increase in disease in people. According to Texas A&M Veterinary Medical Center the rate of cancer in dogs is of particular concern. "35 times more skin cancer, 4 times more breast tumors, 8 times more bone cancer, and twice the incidence of leukemia"

Detoxification protocols, education and awareness are designed to limit the exposure of pollutants and their harmful effects upon the "house" or body. They are now vital and should not be left in the realm of alternative. Animals stand as a warning of what is to come if we do not "Clean House." We are staring at the canary in the coal mine and ignoring its limp body on the bottom of the cage.

BACKYARD
GARAGE
NEIGHBORHOOD,
PARKS, WALKS AND HIKES
TOYS/TREATS
KITCHEN
BATHROOM
BEDROOM
EMOTIONAL TOXICITY
LAUNDRY/UTILITY
LIVING ROOM
OFFICE/DEN
GROOMING
FOOD/WATER
SUPPLEMENTS
VETERINARY CARE
THOUGHTS, WORDS, BELIEFS AS
TOXINS

Notice the Impacts:

Increase in diseases

According to Doris J. Rapp MD, chemical intoxication can change the way you look, behave and even smell. According to Purdue University Department of Veterinary Pathobiology cancer is the second leading cause of death in dogs killing over 25%. Hyperthyroid disease is the leading cause of illness in older cats. Flame retardants (PBDE's) are found at higher levels in cats stricken with this disease. Increases in allergies and auto immune diseases, increases in infections and poor immune systems are responses to our environment.

Behavioral issues

Statistically there is an increase in crime and brutal behavior to each other. "These chemicals can affect learning, behavior (aggression, fatigue, hyperactivity, etc.), fertility and conceivably even parenting and mating behavior." (Rapp PG. 153) There is an increase in cognitive disorders and behavioral problems like anxiety and hyperactivity in pets also.

16

CHAPTER THREE: CHECK LIST -- What to Look for

Check and investigate the ingredient lists and sources of self-poisoning. Notice with in each area of concern other possibilities and add to my lists so you can further educate us pet lovers.

PART 1: Backyard

Example	1 Chemical	1 Impact / Another Straw
Round up/weed killers	Glyphosate	organ damage
		Enzymes shut down
Nitrogen laden fertilizers	Ammonia	endocrine disruptors
	Pesticides	carcinogenicity
Biting Insect Spray	POP's	digestive & nervous system
	Chlordane	
Rodent killers	Warferin	Bleeding
Backyard Burning	Dioxin	carcinogen,
		Endocrine disruptor
Swimming pool/spa	Chlorine	skin, ears, choking etc
Run off poop and pee	Disease	non potable water
Folding chairs	Vinyl	cancer, asthma,
		Hormone disruptor
Garden hoses	Phthalates	neurologic, hormone disruptor
	BPA	
	Heavy Metals	

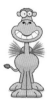

Non Potable Water

Unsafe for human consumption! Ok for lawns. Contain bacteria, coliforms, E.coli, nitrates, herbicides, and pesticides.

This is good for recycling efforts but concentrates over and over chemical run off into non-potable water and eventually into ground water, plants and then animals that eat and drink from them. If you won't drink it, WHY let your pets drink it?

Water Contamination

Often ground water is most contaminated with run off and contains large amounts of pharmaceuticals, animal waste, and chemicals. Often sprinkler systems contain fertilizers and pesticides chemicals for distribution when the grass is watered. Sometimes the system can be hooked up to a non-potable water system. DO NOT LET YOUR PET DRINK FROM THE SPRINKLER.

Animals are at greater risk

They run around the yard naked, don't bathe after and often eat and drink things in the yard. Keeping a "All natural" lawn is even more

important with pets.

PART 2:   Garage

Example	One Chemical	One Impact /Another Straw
Anti-freeze	Ethylene Glycol	severe organ damage & death
Motor oils	Heavy Metals Hydro-carbons	nerve and kidney damage TTCC
Batteries	sulfuric acid, lead	severe burns, blindness, TTCC
Windshield washer fluid	Methanol	organ damage
	Ethylene glycol	organ damage, death
	Isopropanol	irritates, drowsiness, death
Paint	organic solvents	irritates, fatigue, VOC's
Degreasers	Methyl ethyl ketone	Respiratory distress, vertigo,
	Acetone	destroys cell membranes
	Toluene	GI damage and shut down
	Glycolethers	

Heat or cold exposure   **"NEVER leave your pet in the garage"**

VOC

Volatile Organic Compound According to the EPA these are emitted by a wide array of items and are 10X higher indoors than out. They are thought to cause cancer. (TTCC)

STORAGE

Store these products in a locked raised area preferably outside of the connected buildings and rooms of the home you live in. Between temperature changes and concentrated chemicals garage chemicals will increase the VOC's of your home. Heat and Cold is not the only excess exposure in a garage.

Remember a garage is no place to store a pet.

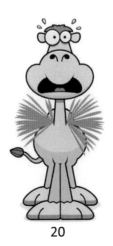

PART 3:   Neighborhood, Parks, Walks and Hikes

Example	One Chemical	One Impact/Another Straw
Sun block	Parabens	hormone disruption (HD)
Cheese dip can lined	BPA	hormone disruption
Plastic bowl	BPA	hormone disruption
Plastic toys	Vinyl	cancer, asthma, HD
Mobile phone	EMF, heavy metals, PVC, BFR's	neurological harm
Insect repellent	DEET	neurologic harm
Vinyl picnic table covers	Phthalates, lead	neuro and endocrine
Vinyl totes, coolers and bags	Vinyl	cancer, asthma, HD
Grass – Pesticides	Fertilizers (via sprinklers)	non-potable water Neuro, HD, TTCC
Styrofoam plates and cups	Styrene	cancer
Water toys	Vinyl	cancer, asthma, HD
Folding chairs	Vinyl	cancer, asthma, HD
Garden hoses	Phthalates BPA, Heavy Metals	neurologic, HD

OMG what did you eat?

	Chem &/ or Biological	GI upset or worse

DEA = DIETHANOLAMINE/TEA
TOBACCO
PROPYLENE GLYCOL
PROPANEDIOL   PABA
SLS/SLE
FLUORIDE
TALC
CHLORINE   ON & ON

ACIDS & ALKALI
ALCOHOL
ALUMINUM
SYNTHETIC FRAGRANCE AND DYES
PARABENS
HEAVY METALS
TRICOLSAN
PESTICIDES AND
FUNGICIDES
PHTHALATES
PETROCHEMICALS
FORMALDEHYDE
SYNTHETIC PRESERVATIVES
MINERAL OIL
CETEARETH-20

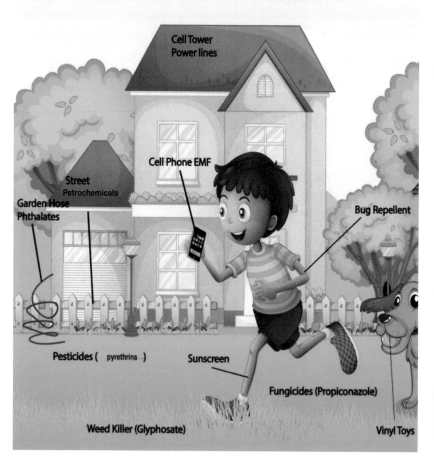

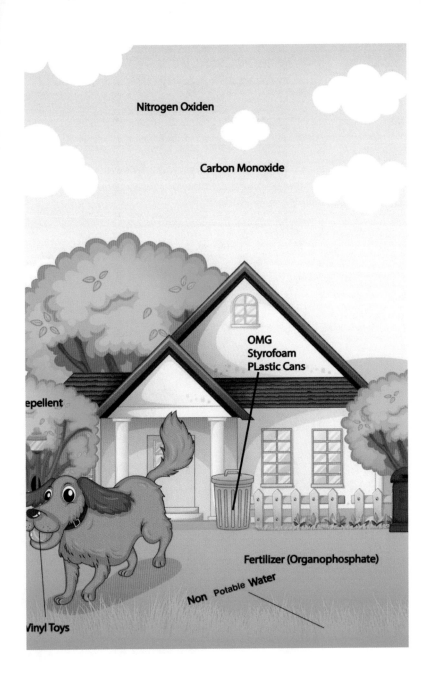

Laundry Room
Fabric Softner
Dry Cleaning
Chlorine/Bleach
Laundry Detergent
Cleaning Products

Outside
Walk in yard
Weed Killer
Pesticides
Fertilizer

25

Bathroom
Air Freshener
Body Wash
Soap
Shampoo and Conditioner
Skin cream and lotion
Shaving Cream and After Shave
Hair Spray

Bedroom
Mattress and Pillows
Pet Bed
Cologne and Perfume
Electronic EMF

Kitchen
Plastic Dishes
Pet Food Packaging
Pet Treats
Pet Supplments
Pet Toothpaste

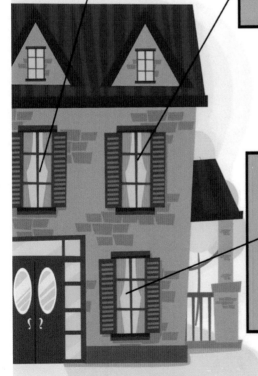

PART 4: KITCHEN

Example	One Chemical	One Impact/Another Straw
Dishwashing detergents	Cationic anionic Nonionic	nausea, vomiting, shock, convulsions, coma, and VOC
	Phosphate	irritant
Automatic dishwasher detergents	same	
Oven cleaners	Lye	extremely corrosive, burns, fatal if swallowed, inhalation damages mucus membranes
Antibacterial soap/cleaners Detergents	Ammonia Lye	
	Cresol	corrosive, damage to liver, kidney, lung and spleen/pancrease
	Phenol	Central Nervous System, depression, affect circulatory system, corrosive, TTCC
	Pine oil	Irritate
Window/ glass cleaners	Ammonia Isopropanol	
Insect bait traps	Organophosphates Carbamates	
Microwaves	EMF pollution	devitalized nutrition

Over the last 30 years, the science and research has come a long way to understand how microwaves affect proteins, antioxidants, and overall nutrient content of food. We've also learned how many toxins flood our food when zapped in the packaging. Today we shouldn't be surprised by these dangers. Instead of microwaving, stick to raw foods as the primary aspect of your diet. When you do cook, try steaming and baking as your main cooking methods.

Washing of food and processing food with chemicals

If you are using water you won't even drink, using cleaning chemicals that you would not want to ingest on food, you are about to eat you are self intoxicating. Water alone will not remove the myriad of petrochemicals adhered to our food these days. You need to wash with clean water with essential oils added to it to fully remove both aqueous and non-aqueous materials. Plants are sprayed with materials that are designed to not wash off in the rain or irrigation system.

Poison people food

List of foods pets should not have

Alcohol, Avocado pit, Chocolate, Coffee, Caffeine, Citrus, Grapes and Raisins, Large amounts of Garlic, Moldy food, Excess Fats, Milk products, Macadamia Nuts, Onions, Xylitol, Apple seeds, Apricot, Cherry or Peach Pits, Leaves and Stems of Potato, Tomato and Rhubarb

PART 5: Bathroom

Anti-bacterial soaps

As the FDA recently noted, antibacterial products are no more effective than soap and water, and could be dangerous.

OTC Triclosan was never fully evaluated by FDA & Triclosan now in wipes, hand gels, cutting boards, mattress pads etc.

1. Target bacteria not viruses

2. Create antibiotic resistant bacteria

3. Endocrine disruptors

4. Higher incidence of development of allergies

5. Bad for the Environment

6. Build up in Fatty tissues

Alternative scrub with water for 30 seconds or more and use a drop of essential oil or essential oil chemical free soap.

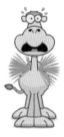

Example	One Chemical	One Impact/Another Straw
Antibacterial soap/cleaner	Tricolosan	HD
Toilet bowel cleaners	Sodium bisulfate	forms sulfuric acid
	Oxalic acid	damage organs, corrodes tissue
	5-dimethyldantoin	forms hypochlorite in water, corrosive
	Hydrochloric acid	burns, extremely corrosive
	Phenol	see above

Leave in toilet bowel cleaners are non-safe for pets to drink, contaminates water and horrible for the environment

Mold & mildew	Chlorine	Respiratory distress
Removers	Alkyl ammonium	burns
	Chlorides	burns
Drain cleaners	Lye	burns
	Sulfuric acid	blindness, corrosive

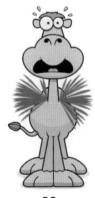

30 Ways we Poison our Pets and Ourselves Before Breakfast

Mattress/pillow	Pet bed
Air freshener products	Bath and Body wash
Shampoo	Conditioner
Skin cream/lotion	Shaving cream
After shave lotion	Skin medications
Face moisturizers and treatments Antiperspirant/deodorant	
Cologne/perfume	Hair spray/products
Toothpaste	Mouthwash
Body Deodorant products	Plastic dishes
Laundry detergent	Fabric softeners
Chlorine bleach	Dry Clean clothes
Cosmetics	Nail polish/Tobacco
Electronic EMF pollution	Pet treat
Pet food material	Pet food packaging
Supplements with fillers	Cleaners
Swimming in Chemicals	

Personal grooming Products   (50% are known carcinogens)

Medications

List of human OTC products toxic to pets

According to Pet Poison Help Line and the AVMA

1. NSAIDS

2. Acetaminophen

3. Antidepressants

4. ADD/ADHD medication

5. Sleep aids / Antianxiolytics

6. Birth control pill

7. ACE inhibitors

8. Beta Blockers

9. Thyroid hormones

10. Statins

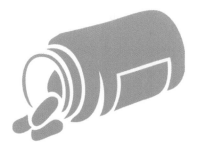

Pets can eat through bottles and baggies. Never leave loose pills out on own or in baggies. Store pills, powders and creams out of reach especially in a suitcase. Never store your medication with your pet's medications, often mistakes can happen. Hang your purse or bag up away from pets especially when visiting a home with pets. Ask visitors to place their items up out of your pets reach.

Phthalates

"Phthalates are hormone-disrupting chemicals that can be particularly dangerous for young children and unborn babies. Exposure to phthalates can affect testosterone levels and lead to reproductive abnormalities, including abnormal genitalia and reduced sperm production. The State of California notes that five types of phthalates -- including one that we found in air freshener products -- are 'known to cause birth defects or reproductive harm.'"

-- Natural Resources Defense Council

PART 6: BEDROOM

Fire Retardants

Firefighters are actively trying to get toxic flame retardants banned from furniture, saying that they make home fires much more dangerous to family members and fire fighters when they breathe the toxic fumes during the fire. According to National Center for Health Research

Toxic flame-retardants are used in upholstered furniture such as couches, chairs, and mattresses, including infant crib mattresses, and in drapery and carpets. Flame retardants have also been found in the foam inside baby products such as baby carriers, high chairs, strollers, and nursing pillows.

Some flame retardants are made of chemicals called volatile or semi-volatile organic compounds (VOCs or SVOCs), which simply means that they can become airborne or collect on the dust particles we breathe.

1.   Contribute to the VOC content of home

2.   Endocrine disruptors and neuro disruptors

3.   TTCC

4.   Accumulate in house dust

5.   Mattress, pillows and bedding, furniture and plastic housing Units

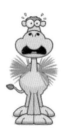

These are all the places our pets lay around on naked for hours. They breathe it in all day long, they ingest as they clean themselves and it is absorbed through their skin and, as they do not bathe daily, it accumulates and concentrates. This happens all night and day long!!

Example	One Chemical	One Impact/Another Straw
Dry cleaning	Perchloroethylene	Registered as toxic air pollutant by EPA dizziness, headache, neuro depression
Moth balls	Naphthalene P-dichlorobenzene	
Mattress/pillows	Fire retardants Chlorinated tris	VOC's TTCC
Air fresheners	contribute to VOC	TTCC

The Natural Resources Defense Council studied the effects of air fresheners, discovering that they currently undergo no safety testing. The results were disturbing, because they revealed high levels of phthalates, which are known to be especially harmful to children and even more so for pets. These chemicals were even present in sprays that were claimed to be "All-Natural" and "unscented". Phthalates were not disclosed in the list of ingredients for any of the products.

PART 7: LAUNDRY/UTILITY

Phosphates

Harmful to the Environment
Recycling our toxins accumulating and concentrating
to lethal levels killing our Water ways
10% of all toxic exposure is Phosphates in the ground water.

"Get over the water spots. If they bother you, wipe them off with
a towel. New products can butt heads with our old cultural
concepts of cleanliness. As I see it, we all need to start making
some concessions for the good of our planet and our health."
Mercola

Our solution is we must change our standards from those of
convenience to those of earth friendly standards of cleanliness.

Chloramme Gas

Made by mixing ammonia and chlorine

DEADLY – Never mix cleaning products

Issue with Fragrance

Environmental Working Group researchers found more than
75 percent of products listing the ingredient "fragrance"
contained phthalates (THAL-ates) which have been shown
to disrupt hormone activity, reduce sperm counts, and
cause reproductive malformation, and have been linked to
liver and breast cancer, diabetes, and obesity. Additionally,
studies by Dr. Philip J. Landrigan of the Mount Sinai
Children's Environmental Health Center, link fetal exposure
with autism, ADHD, and neurological disorders.

Laundry detergent

SURFACTANTS

PETROLEUM DISTILLATES
(NAPHTHAS)

LINEAR
ALKYL SODIUM SULFONATES
(LAS) ANIONIC

PHENOIS
OPTICAL BRIGHTENERS

SODIUM HYPOCHLORITE

EDTA

ARTIFICIAL FRAGRANCES OR
POOR QUALITY NATURAL
FRAGRANCES

Example	One Chemical	One Impact/Another Straw
All purpose cleaners	Ammonia Fumes	irritate tissues burns rashes
	Ethylene Glycol Poison	damage to organs dizziness
	Sodium Hypochlorite	corrosive damage to organ
Bleach	Sodium Hypochlorite solution	corrosive damage to organs
Dryer sheets	biodegradable cationic softeners	havoc on nervous system

Fabric softener

According to the health and wellness website Sixwise.com, some of the
most harmful ingredients in dryer sheets and liquid fabric softener alike
include benzyl acetate (linked to pancreatic cancer), benzyl alcohol (an
upper respiratory tract irritant), ethanol (linked to central nervous
system disorders), limonene (a known carcinogen) and chloroform (a
neurotoxin and carcinogen), among others.

Pet Flea and Tick Treatments /Supplies

On all of these the EPA have found considerable health risks.

They are managed under the EPA as they are all considered pesticides.

Example	One Chemical	One Impact/Another Straw
Insecticides	see garden area	
Household foggers	see veterinary area for full details	
Weed killers	diquat,2,4-D,	skin and eye irritant, Central Nervous System disturbance
	Glyphosate	abdominal pain, nausea, vomiting & diarrhea

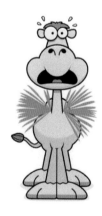

PART 8: Living Room

Green home products

The FDA does not regulate the term "natural".

Many Marketing techniques use "Green" or the perception of "Green" to sell us more products:

Association marketing such as:

"We give to the Sierra Club" therefore we should believe it to be Natural by the message.

Ask who is the owner of the company and what is their end game?

Market research showed:

Consumers are put off by "fragrance free" stating that the smell tells them it is clean They perceive it as less clean if they do not smell lots of fragrance.

Change your standard now to "less chemical equals more clean" and don't be a lemming and go with what market research says.

Marketing ploy of mincing words like:

Organic alcohol is still alcohol so look for 100% biodegradable alcohol free instead

Careful not to contribute to the drive of mass consumerism:

Mass waste and consumption comes from all these "Go Green" new products

Truly going green is not buying the new gadgets that advocate Green is easier. Part of going green is to reduce consumerism. Green initiatives go beyond renewable energy and recycling and MUST be non-consumerism focused. Instead of feeding the non-sustainable Billon dollar green business stop where you are, turn off lights, protest for change by hosting a party to promote chemical free lifestyles and don't buy anything for a year; Or at least ignore the message to buy more to save the planet, instead consume less and support sustainable development.

Example	One Chemical	One Impact/Another Straw
Rug and carpet upholstery cleaners	Perchloroethylene	VOC, dizziness, sleepiness nausea, disorientation TTCC
	Naphthalene	liver damage, eye
Furniture Polish	Ammonia, Paphitha, Nitrobenzene, Petroleum	
	Distillates Phenol	Irritate tissues, nausea, vomiting
Air fresheners	Formaldehyde Petroleum	strong irritant TTCC
	Distillates	Strong irritant, Fatal pulmonary edema, Flammable
	P-Dichlorobenzene	irritation
	Aerosol propellants	brain damage, highly flammable
	Cigarettes	air pollution, known to cause cancer allergies, resp issues weakened immune behavior issues

Correlation found between skin exposure and disease like allergies and cancer.

Tobacco & Pets

In addition to inhaling carcinogens, your smoking habit can harm pets in some surprising ways:

By ingesting cigarette or cigar butts, which contain high levels of nicotine and other toxins

By drinking water that contains cigar or cigarette butts, where nicotine has become concentrated

By ingesting nicotine replacement gum and patches, or cigarettes, cigars or snuff

The toxic level of nicotine, for both dogs and cats, is 0.5-1.0 mg of nicotine per pound of body weight. In dogs, 10 mg/kg is *potentially fatal.*

One cigarette contains 15-25 mg of nicotine, depending on the brand. The butt of a cigarette has a surprisingly large concentration of nicotine for its size -- 4 to 8 mg.

Signs and symptoms of nicotine poisoning in your dog or cat include:

Tremors, twitching, or seizures

Drooling Constricted pupils

Auditory and visual hallucinations

Excitement, racing heart (but slow heart rate with small doses)

Vomiting and diarrhea

Published studies in the 1970's and yet are still sold and smoked

20 years after first Surgeon General's report before any government action was taken

E-Cigs/Vaping dangers include eating the capsule, and inhalation. Poisoning from nicotine and propylene glycol. Inhaling vegetable oil may set up reactions in lung tissues and contribute to respiratory issues and cancer.

Nicotine gum	contain xylitol and nicotine
Fire retardants	see previous
TDCIPPs	disrupt endocrine system
Television	dust collects VOC, EMF pollution (see box)

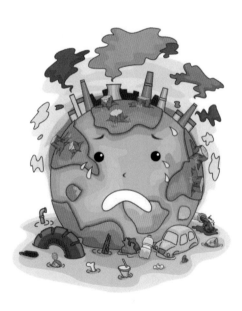

Diffuser Advantage

Diffusing essential oils into the air of your home is a great way for everyone to experience the benefits of essential oils! And if that isn't reason enough, try this ...conventional room deodorizers that you plug into your wall or leave on your table top contain up to 37% formaldehyde! Ditch your conventional fresheners and opt for ultrasonic diffuser for emotional oils such as *Pelargonium graveolenos* or *Lavendula angustifolia*. Choose a nebulizing diffuser for the most powerful benefits with oils such as *Cinnamomum zeylanicum or Syzygiuma aromaticum*

Know your Environment --- Protect your Health

Safe4animals.com for even more information

EPA 7x more pollution indoor vs outdoor 100x more due to cleaners alone

PART 9: Office/Den

EMF Pollution

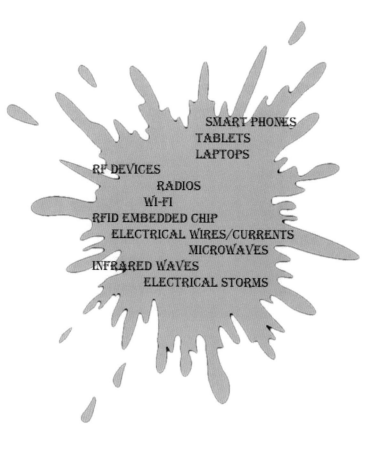

SMART PHONES
TABLETS
LAPTOPS
RF DEVICES
RADIOS
WI-FI
RFID EMBEDDED CHIP
ELECTRICAL WIRES/CURRENTS
MICROWAVES
INFRARED WAVES
ELECTRICAL STORMS

Dirty Electricity

Too many electromagnetic fields surrounding us—from cell phones, Wi-Fi, and commonplace modern technology— may be seriously harming our health.

In 2007, the Bio initiative Working Group, an international collaboration of prestigious scientists and public health policy experts from the United States, Sweden, Denmark, Austria, and China, released a 650-page report citing more than 2,000 studies (many very recent) that detail the toxic effects of EMFs from all sources. Chronic exposure to even low-level radiation (like that from cell phones), the scientists concluded, can cause a variety of cancers, impair immunity, and contribute to Alzheimer's disease and dementia, heart disease, and many other ailments. "We now have a critical mass of evidence, and it gets stronger every day," says David Carpenter, MD, director of the Institute for Health and the Environment at the University at Albany and coauthor of the public-health chapters of the Bio initiative report.

Exposure to electromagnetic fields is not a new phenomenon.

However, during the 20th century, environmental exposure to man-made electromagnetic fields has been steadily increasing as growing electricity demand, ever-advancing technologies and changes in social behavior have created more and more artificial sources. Everyone is exposed to a complex mix of weak electric and magnetic fields, both at home and at work, from the generation and transmission of electricity, domestic appliances and industrial equipment, to telecommunications and broadcasting.

Tiny electrical currents exist in the human body due to the chemical reactions that occur as part of the normal bodily functions, even in the absence of external electric fields. For example, nerves relay signals by transmitting electric impulses. Most biochemical reactions from digestion to brain activities go along with the rearrangement of charged particles. Even the heart is electrically active - an activity that your doctor can trace with the help of an electrocardiogram.

PART 10: Grooming

Example   One Chemical   One Impact/Another Straw

Perfumes   See Fragrance and VOC's

Cleaners   See Kitchen, laundry and bathroom

Shampoo   See Personal Care section bathroom

Conditioner

Emotional

Stress is the number one cause of acid to build up in the body; sugar is a close second. Self-intoxication can be made from the byproducts of maintaining a flight or fight response for hours while at a place a pet cannot relax. Train your pet to love the groomer. Switch groomers, use mobile groomers. Respect your pets fear and counter condition them so they do not build as much toxic waste in their body as if they were just dumped into a vat of chemicals. See Dr. Nancy book "Are We Helping Our Pets?"

Noise

Have you ever had a car pull up next to you and the booming of the bass came through. Could you ignore it or did your attention get drawn to it? Noise to pets is exactly the same. They are programmed to be alerted to change in their environment and be on alert until they know what to do about the noise.   Noise is not just irritating; we have known for some time that it can have direct human health impacts. Indeed, chronic exposure to noise levels above 55dB dramatically increases the risks of heart disease and stroke.

SLS – Sodium Lauryl Sulfate

SLES – Sodium Laureth Sulfate

Used as a Surfactant

Studies to induce mutations in bacteria

Skin irritant, mutagenesis

Corrodes hair follicles and impairs hair re-growth

Binds with nitrates to form carcinogens

Residual levels in the heart, liver, lungs and brain found via skin contact

Denatures protein

Impairs eye maturity

Damage skin level immunity

Sublingual absorption very powerful

Bypasses liver protection

In toothpaste and mouth washes

Warning on toothpaste to not swallow it and if you do contact poison control

Cannot sue because they have warned you

SLS found in nearly all toothpastes, shampoos and bubble baths

Absorbed through skin and retained for 5 days

Increase rate of glasses and contacts

Long term consequences not high dose short term that matter to us

"Studies are skewed and dated"

PART 11: Food/Water

Pet food recalls

A food recall occurs when there is reason to believe that a food may cause consumers to become ill. A food manufacturer or distributor initiates the recall to take foods off the market. In some situations, food recalls are requested by government agencies (USDA or FDA).

Some reasons for recalling food include:

- Discovery of an organism in a product which may make consumers sick
- Discovery of a potential allergen in a product
- Mislabeling or misbranding of food. For example, a food may contain an allergen, such as nuts or eggs, but those ingredients do not appear on the label.

Food recalls typically involve only a limited number of product runs and batches. So, just because a specific recipe has been recalled does not mean the entire brand should be considered defective.

Unless they become a habit, individual manufacturing accidents should not be interpreted as a sign of an inferior producer.

Recalls are usually voluntary. Sometimes a company discovers a problem and recalls a product on its own. Other times, a company recalls a product after the FDA raises concerns. Only rarely will the FDA order a recall.

A dog food can be recalled for almost any reason. A few of the most common causes include contamination with mold, bacteria (like Salmonella) or a toxic substance (like aflatoxin).

The Triple Whammy Food Chain

GMO corn contains more than 18X the "safe" level of glyphosate set by the EPA. Our pets are not only exposed to weed killer via a walk in the park, via skin and inhalation, often it is the number one ingredient in their pet food!

Triple Whammy:

1. The chemical – Glyphosate – is on lawns and gains contact via skin, allowed to accumulate and concentrate, and promotes absorption through the skin or licked off and ingested or both.

2. The Chemical – Glyphosate – is found concentrated in ground water and run-off water and may be inhaled, ingested or dermally absorbed.

3. It is concentrated in the food our pets eat. The cows or chickens eat the GMO corn with 18X the safe level so it concentrates in their meat and then to add injury to insult we add GMO corn as a main ingredient to their processed food. Our pets are getting it from all ways to Sunday.

Example	One Chemical	One Impact/Another Straw
Cans, pouches, dishes	Aluminum	Metal and a toxin processed foods, antiperspirants, antacids, cosmetics, paper products, beverage cans, foil and cookware., and water treatment plants.
Toxic plastics	Bisphenol-A	alter behavior of over 200 genes

Alzheimer's link high concentrations of Aluminum in brain

4th leading cause of DEATH

50 years ago the disease did not exists.

We are seeing significant rises in Cognitive Disorder in pets also.

Drinking water supply

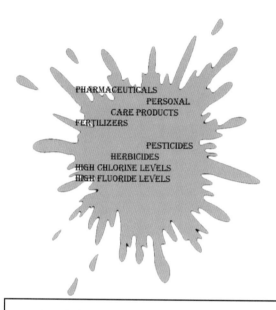

PHARMACEUTICALS
PERSONAL
CARE PRODUCTS
FERTILIZERS

PESTICIDES
HERBICIDES
HIGH CHLORINE LEVELS
HIGH FLUORIDE LEVELS

EPA finds 202 unregulated chemicals in 45 states

The Environmental Working Group analysis of 20 million tap water quality tests found a total of 316 contaminants -- including industrial solvents, weed killers, refrigerants and the rocket fuel component perchlorate -- in water supplied to the public between 2004 and 2009.

Pet food:

AFLATOXINS (MYCOTOXINS)
PROPYLENE GLYCOL
ANTIBIOTIC RESISTANT BACTERIA
ETHOXYQUIN   RANCID FATS
BUTYLATED HYDROXYANISOLE (BHA)
TBHQ
PROPYL GALLATE
BUTYLATED HYDROXYTOLENE (BHT)
BENZOIC ACID
SODIUM BENZOATE
POTASSIUM BENZOATE
SODIUM NITRATE
SODIUM NITRITE
TOCOPHENOLS
CARRAGEENAN
CONTAMINATES   PRESERVATIVES
MINERAL OIL
PABA   CETEARETH-20
GLYPHOSATE
EUTHANASIA SOLUTION

Need I say more?

See book **"Evolutionary Feeding of Pets"**
www.safe4animals.com

PART 12: Treats

If they appeal to you and you want to eat them then they were marketed to you, not for your carnivore. Treats should be meat and not look like cute bones made out of cracker material. Treats should be bendable not hardened pieces of tanned hide. Some treats are treated with multiple chemical washes to appeal to the consumer – HUMAN – and yet our pets are the ones consuming them. Would you soak your meat in ammonia and bleach solution prior to eating it? Many treats contain dyes to appeal to – Humans – thinking they should be brightly colored and look like a little piece of dyed meat product even though it is a piece of cracker material. Would you feed your child chips as their only form of side dish?

Many treats are treated with chemicals to prevent decay so they can be packaged and put on a shelf instead of refrigerated this kills all raw enzymes and probiotics and leaves residues which will then kill good bacteria in our pets gut and limit their immune and digestive function. See more in Dr. Nancy's book **"Evolutionary Feeding of Pets"**

Plastic dishes   Breed bacteria

Pieces break off and cause irritation of the mouth and gums

If swallowed irritation of GI system

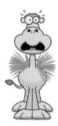

PART 13: Supplements

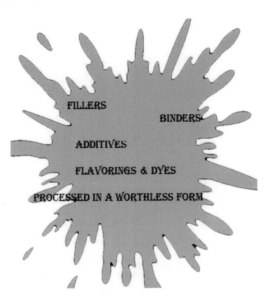

FILLERS

BINDERS

ADDITIVES

FLAVORINGS & DYES

PROCESSED IN A WORTHLESS FORM

Whole Food Live Food

Just like refined foods, these refined vitamins have been robbed of all of the extra accessory nutrients that they naturally come with as well. In turn, like refined foods, they can create numerous problems and imbalances in your body if taken at high levels for long periods of time. They can also act more like drugs in your body, forcing themselves down one pathway or another. At the very least, they won't help you as much as high quality food.

Take a Carrot for Instance.

Carrots are loaded with nutrients. Bigwigs like beta-carotene (a precursor to vitamin A) and ascorbic acid (vitamin C), as well as lesser-known players like folicin and mannose. In fact, scientists have isolated about 200 nutrients and phytonutrients in the humble carrot.

These 200 nutrients work together in mysterious ways. The little guys help get the big guys and vice versa, There are enzymes, coenzymes, co-vitamins , minerals, and other factors that help the nutrients work together synergistically.

Scientists don't know how all this works, and they probably never will. It's the magic and mystery of nature. Foods are complex in their nutrients because nutrients need each other to be properly absorbed and integrated into our bodies.

Whole-food whiz Judith DeCava, CNC, LNC writes in her book *The Real Truth About Vitamins and Antioxidants*:

Natural food concentrates will show a much lower potency in milligrams or micrograms. This is frequently interpreted to mean they are less effective, not as powerful. Unfortunately, the `more is better' philosophy is far from nutritional truth.

Simply put, if the vitamin concentrations are high and/or their natural sources aren't listed, most likely these vitamins are synthetic. Chemical sources for synthetic vitamin supplements include petrochemicals, coal tar, chemically manipulated sugar and inorganic minerals

Toys are mentally and physically stimulating and assist in fulfilling a dog's emotional and physical needs. Even though dogs today are primarily bred as companion pets, they still need something to do. In the absence of a "job", they will look for things to do to occupy their time and fulfill their chewing needs. If you don't want them to choose their own chew toys, such as your sofa, pillows, shoes, or toilet paper rolls, provide them with appropriate chemical free outlets.

PART 14: Toys

What else to look out for:

Latex

Nylon

Plastic

Cleaners

Synthetic materials

Dyes

Very hard quiet toys are dangerous and boring

Very soft toys or toys that pieces come off easily are

dangerous and are a choking or GI blockage risk

Toys that appeal to you cute and cuddly are not safe

Toys that are a dime a dozen are not safe

Toys that can be swallowed and become a choke or digestive hazard can lead to 10% or more of pets deaths a year.

Lobby for warning labels to be placed on toys or treats that are unsafe.

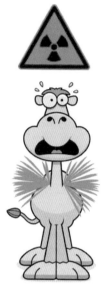

Best toys – natural raw meaty bones of appropriate size and shape. Do not feed unless you have read "Evolutionary Feeding of Pets"

Toys should fulfill your pet's psychological needs.

1. Toys are like prey to a pet. The endgame: taste great, smell great. can be torn apart and make noise.
2. Want toys that mimic a captured prey body and the excitement of the hunt.
3. Want new things, the endgame are hunt, capture, devour NEXT.
4. Social animals want to hunt together. Engaging a pet in play with toys is much more of an adventure and will encourage rest and relaxation after the meal.

PART 15: Veterinary Care

Restraint -- Respect and Honor Boundaries

Rats laugh in response to being tickled. Chimpanzees mourn their dead. Dogs jump and wag their tails when they see a familiar face. These are just a few examples of animals' sentience, their ability to feel pleasure and pain and to be aware of their surroundings. In all probability, they represent the tip of a neurobehavioral iceberg. That is, animals have sensory and cognitive capacities that we are only now beginning to appreciate. And these capacities suggest that many ways that humans treat animals need to be rethought, in light of animals' capacity to suffer.

Ever wonder what happens when your pet is taken in the back? Ask to go with your pet. Ever wonder what goes through your pets mind when they are restrained and asked to expose a vessel and let a stranger puncture it to remove blood? Is it possible your pet is in fear?

How Veterinary personnel interact with your pet during visits is just as important as how they clean their place or if they do "Holistic Medicine". If the staff are in a hurry and carry urgent energy your pet is going to think there is danger and get in a heightened state of awareness. Make sure the people you choose to treat your pets use respectful, safe humane restraint and honor your pet's boundaries without harm to themselves or others.

A pet does not kick, bite or scratch because they are hunting their next meal or mean they do so because energetically they feel threatened.

More about this in **"Are We Helping Our Pets?"** by Dr. Nancy

Cancer Rates

1900	1 in 80
1950	1 in 20
1975	1 in 3
2010	1 in 1.5

Cancer is not a foreign invader. It is a self-defense mechanism against a storm of toxins the body was not designed to fight.

Increase Toxic Factors

Cleaning products	see previous
Air fresheners	see previous
Noise	see previous
Stress	see previous
Rushed Energy	see previous
Smells	200,000x more powerful than our own sense of smell
Vaccinations	research now shows less is better
Antibiotics	research now shows less is better & alternatives may be better
Heartworm preventative	see Pet Flea and Tick
Flea & Tick preventative	see Pet Flea and Tick

Surgeries

Is Anesthetic more toxic than fear? Studies show that the toxic effects of fear in some animals can lead to death. Sedation and Anesthetics are as much for the pet's wellbeing as they are to create restraint and pain management.

Blood work

This often can catch things earlier.   Doing yearly blood work gives the veterinarian a comparison and they can notice trends and changes. When we catch dis-ease early often it can be reversed or slowed to increase our pets quality and quantity of life.

XRays/Ultrasound

Often extremely helpful in finding out answers or even eliminating a cause. Ask am I doing a procedure to help myself or my pet? Ask will the answers I find by this procedure change the treatment protocol

Chronic medication and over medicating our pets is becoming the number one cause of toxicity in pets. Ask am I medicating my pet to control normal behaviors that I am not willing to use training and together time to manage? Are their alternative treatments to lessen medication needs like Acupuncture or Manipulation techniques to lessen pain medication use? Many Alternatives are discussed in "First Aid using Veterinary Medical Aromatherapy" and "Safe and Effective Veterinary Medical Aromatherapy"

Western Medicine is our friend!! Do not avoid a veterinarian because you want to stay chemical free. Seek a veterinarian who is utilizing as many ways to be chemical free as possible and yet still knows that sometimes the best tool in the tool box is the western, conventional, regular medicine tool. You cannot be "Whole-istic" while throwing away western medicine. Utilize it asking more questions and demanding with your voting dollar they also support a Go Green initiative.

Always ask: What is the Risk? What is the Benefit?

Pet Flea and Tick

Example treatments/ supplies	One Chemical	One Impact/Another Straw
		Of all of these the EPA have found considerable health risks. They are managed under the EPA as they are all considered pesticides
Insecticides	Butopyronoxyl	necrosis of liver
	Cimethyl Phthalate	CNS damage
	Diethyltoluamide (DEET)	irritate respiratory tract
		loss of coordination anxiety behavioral issues and outbursts
Household fogger	Pyrethrins	severe allergic dermatitis
		systemic allergic reactions
		CNS disturbances
		nausea, vomiting
		headache, tinnitus
	Permethrin	itching burning skin
		URT and eye irritation
	Methoprene	skin and eye irritant
	Fipronil	nervous and thyroid toxicity
		liver and kidney toxicity
		decrease fertility and convulsions
	Imidacloprid	thyroid lesions, liver toxicity, organ damage
		neurotoxin
	Pyrethroids	brain damage,
		heart disease, seizures
	Permethrin	lung cancer, liver tumors, neurotoxin,
		tremors, aggression, endocrine disruption

List of toxic essential oils for pets

Most essential oils are quite safe especially if used appropriately and are a clean Biologicaly Active® essential oils (see book Biologically Active® Essential Oils)

Most essential oils can cause harm and even death if used inappropriately. If they are altered or synthetic poorly processed oils they ARE TOXIC Chemicals - PERIOD!!!

Many uses and oils are discussed in "First Aid using Veterinary Medical Aromatherapy®" and "Safe and Effective Veterinary Medical Aromatherapy" by Dr. Nancy

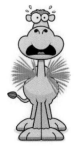

Here is the short list:

In birds: Dilute significantly 1 drop in 4 ounces of water leave lots of ventilation

Do not use oils for long periods in close confinement with birds unventilated. Avoid hotter oils.

In cats: Dilute 1 drop in 2 ounces of water and leave an escape route. Pets know when they have had enough. Honor their need to escape the diffuser. Avoid hotter oils.

In dogs: Dilute 1 drop in 1 ounce of water. Most oils are safe and effective when used with proper education. Go to safe4animals.com for free videos and classes. Use hot oils with caution.

In horses: Dilute 1 drop in 1 ounce of water. Most oils are safe and effective when used with proper education. Go to   safe4animals.com for free videos and classes. Use hot oils with caution.

Avoid use on eyes. Never apply to inside of ears. Do not allow ingestion unless you know it is a safe oil for ingestion. Never apply to bottom of feet. Never apply if your pet is running for the hills. Their olfactory system is telling them it is the wrong oil, use an alternative. Go to safe4animals.com for videos and classes.

Hot oils:

Cinnamomum zylanicum

Syzyqium aromaticum

Cybopogon flexuosus

Melaleuca alternifolia

Oreganum Vulgare

Mentha piperita

Thymus vulgris

Gaultheria procumbens

Cinnamomum Cassia

Acorus calamus

Zingiber officinale

Curcuma longa

Piper nigrum

Rosmarinus officinalis

Avoid when you can:

CO2 extractions

Absolute extractions

Cross reactions when applying more than one oil over the top of another

Possible Toxic oils:

Cinnamomum camphora

Sassafras albidum

Ocotea cymbarum

Thuja occidentalis

Artemisia absinthium

Turpentine

Advise Careful use:

Pimpinella anisum

Ocimum basilicum

Syzygium aromaticum

Coriandrum sativum

Hyssopus officinalis

Salvia officinalis

Colophony resina

Angelica archangelica

Citrus aurantium bergamia

Cinannamomum Cassia

Cumium cyminun

Get educated on using essential oils with pets.
www.safe4animals.com

PART 16: Emotional Toxicity

The emotional climate your pet must live in day in and day out is just as toxic as stress and chemicals. Be mindful of how you emit energy around your pets. Look at "Are We Helping Our Pets?" book by Dr. Nancy for more info

PART 17: Thoughts, words, beliefs as toxins

The same for emotions all words thoughts and beliefs carry a energy signal that can impact our pets just like EMF's can impact them. Positive thoughts words and beliefs go a far way to support our pet's health. Look at **"Are We Helping Our Pets?"** book by Dr. Nancy

Is it too late?

NO – utilize detoxification programs and support the waste management systems of the body.

See book by Dr. Nancy called

"The 4 Pillars of Health"

CHAPTER FOUR : When to Look for Chemicals

Birth to 8 weeks   Chemical free breeder

No vaccinations before 12-16 weeks

Raw food

Stay with Mom until 8 weeks at least

Mom and litter tested for immunity
rather than vax

8 weeks to 16 weeks   Homeward to a forever home

Commit

1st vax 12 weeks earliest,

2nd vax 16 weeks

Training is for us to talk "Dog, Horse or Cat". We must learn their language, their behavior, because they are not little people. Seek behavior trainers and Natural Horseman. If there is a tug of war and effort on the trainers part, CHANGE!!

The number one reason animals are put to sleep and surrendered is behavior issues that are failure of Guardians to translate.

16 weeks to 6 months   Spay or neuter put off until later some states
have laws
Chemical free Insect control
Chemical free Veterinarian
Chemical free Groomer
Chemical free walk in the park

<u>6 months to 18 months</u> Consider spay and neuter later around 18 months

Consider sparing ovaries

Continue chemical free

Raw feeding - evolutionary appropriate feeding

Start Chiropractic or strength training

<u>1-5 years</u>
Spay or neuter Debate –
Research supports either choice.
Every 6 months chiropractic
Yearly detoxification programs
Chemical free supplements
Continue evolutionary appropriate feeding

<u>5-10 years</u>
Yearly blood work checks
Every 1-3 months chiropractic
Chemical free supplements
Every 6 months detox program
(see **"The 4 Pillars of Health"** by Dr. Nancy)
Continue evolutionary appropriate feeding

<u>10-15 years</u>
Every 6 months blood work checks
Every month chiropractic
Chemical free supplements
Every 6 months detox program
Continue evolutionary appropriate feeding

<u>15+ years</u>
Once a month fluid therapy
Every 6 months blood work checks
Every month chiropractic
Chemical free supplements
Every 6 months detox program
Continue evolutionary appropriate feeding

List of Go Green Pet Friendly Businesses

and

List of Veterinary Medical Aromatherapy® Trained

Veterinarians on Vmaa.vet

Training and education on Safe4animals.com

Safe essential oils on Safearomatherapy.com

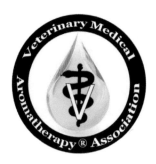

CHAPTER SIX: How to Live Chemical Free

A.   Alternatives & Awareness

With awareness and alternatives it is possible to change the Load or Burden on our pets.

Is it possible to have ZERO contact with chemicals? NO

Is it possible to cut down on the amount of chemicals and toxins in your pet's life time? YES

The most important aspect of shifting the chemical burden of our pets is the choices we make within our own home. There are lots of websites out there with ideas. There are lots of books touching on "Go Green" movements. Know how to find green pet businesses. When "Green" is not an option remember western medicine is our friend just detox!

Host a Party

Train a Guardian

Help a Pet

Save a Planet

Go to safe4animals.com for full instructions

On teaching your friends and family chemical

free lifestyles for their pets.

B. Essential Oils Contribution to a Chemical Free lifestyle

What is an essential Oil?

An essential oil is nature's living energy from a plant which offers its protection, strength and vitality. The volatile liquid extracted from the plant can come from seeds, bark, stems, leaves, flowers, roots, fruit, etc. The seeds used for planting, the time and methods of harvesting , the means of distillation, all impact the purity and potency of the essential oil. The purer the essential oil, the stronger its effects.

The level of biological impact depends on the nature of captured biological activity of the essential oil.

 Only purchase Biologically Active®Essential Oils.

Extraction Methods

There are several different ways from which the essential oils of a plant get from mother nature's source to a bottle. The choice of manufacturers and oils can leave you overwhelmed and walking away empty handed. Educating ourselves about different choices available will leave you with a collection of oils that will deliver the restorative results that you set off in search of. Here are three of the most common practices used today to separate an essential oil. Always remember that different quality oils deliver different results, throughout the extraction processes, the most crucial part of the plants healing components can be lost or severely damaged.

1. Chemical Extraction: Hexane & ethanol are used to extract the essential oil from its plant source. People with chemical sensitivities may have reactions to these oils. Solvent based isolation methods can extract more essential oil/pound of plant source than steam distillation thus making solvent extracted essential oils less expensive to buy. Traces of the solvent chemicals are often found present in the final bottled product.

2. CO2 Extraction: Plant material is placed in a pressure vessel and pumped liquefied gas or solvent at a specific pressure and temperature.
3. Steam distillation: For 1000's of years, distillation has been used to produce essential oils. Ask if your company developed a specialized process that uses extremely low pressure and low temperatures. These specifically designed distillers, constructed of food grade (not ferrous) stainless steel that does not react with essential oils, results in pure 100 percent therapeutic grade essential oils. Ask if your company's plants are harvested and distilled in a manner as to protect every element of nature's power. Does your company have standards that have made them the world leader in essential oils for over 20 years? Always look for Biologically Active® essential oils.

Benefits of Pure Therapeutic oils!

- Maintain your emotional, spiritual and physical health.
- Through clinical research, scientists have discovered that essential oils raise the frequency of a Biological System thus helping it to maintain an optimal level.
- Research has proven that essential oils quickly penetrate through the skin.
- Because of their ability to penetrate through the skin, essential oils can affect the cells of a Biological System within minutes.
- Essential oils are powerful in helping to create an environment unfriendly for free-radicals.
- Essential oils can affect multiple body systems to maintain health and vitality.

(See "Biologically Active® Essential Oils" by Dr. Nancy)

- Essential oils can benefit physical and spiritual well-being. They can be invigorating, relaxing, stimulating, calming, soothing, or uplifting and promote optimal cellular health. (See Biologically Active ®Essential Oils by Dr. Nancy Brandt).
- Various Biologically Active ®Essential Oils can be applied topically, ingested, diffused, or inhaled - therefore, be sure to check your labels for individual details.
- Essential oils containing Sesquiterpenes have the ability to pass the blood brain barrier thus making them effective for optimal daily clarity for cognitive health.
- There are 188 references to essential oils in the Bible
- For thousands of years, rare and valuable plant essential oils were prized for their rejuvenating abilities, often more valuable than gold and only offered to royalty.
- Essential oils afford families the option to take control of their own health and wellness while creating an environment free of toxic chemicals.
- Essential oils play an invaluable role in maintaining wellness from infancy through your golden years. Go to safe4animals.com for more information.

C.   **Going Green on Any Budget**

Green is not trendy. Green is vital to sustaining life on this planet.

Reuse Glass Containers

Wash purchased food containers, Buy Glass Packaged food.

Mason Jars are a cheap alternative to storing in plastic.

Laundry/Bath towels

>
> Hang on the line instead of dryer
> Fluff up with spritzer of white vinegar and
> essential oil of choice
> Then fluff for just a few minutes in the dryer

Plant a Garden

>
> Food containers to plant your starter plants in for your
> garden compost

Eat /buy locally

>
> Locally grown food will reduce your carbon footprint
> (No transport costs or emissions)
> (Eliminate Packing costs)

Go solar

>
> Wherever you can use solar and support Green
> companies that use solar and limit their carbon
> footprint.

Stretch Products

>
> Essential oils are so concentrated that you can add
> water, vodka or Witch hazel to the empty bottle and
> use as spritzers to become air fresheners to use with in
> house, car and body; or use as fabric fresheners.

Recycle – Reuse – Reduce – Repurpose – Buy used

We must reduce our environmental impact. Transform from consumerism to sustainability. Look to Nature as an example of a bio-sustainable cycle of life.

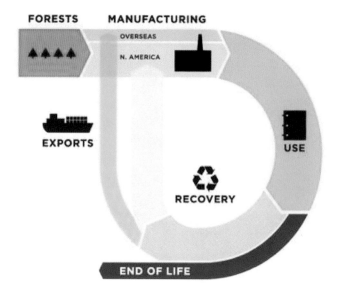

_D. Take 10 steps to Change Your Footprint on the Ecosystem

1. Save energy
2. Save water
3. Use less petrochemicals
4. Eat smart
5. Eliminate plastic especially water bottles
6. Think before you buy
   > Borrow instead of buying
   > Buy smart
   > Repurpose
   > Reuse
   > Buy used
7. Keep electronics out of the trash
8. The more "Raw" the product the less taxing it is on the ecosystem
9. Host parties that teach Awareness
10. Make your own cleaning supplies

1. Save Energy
2-3 degrees change in thermostat

LED light bulbs

"Smart" power strips

Wash in cold water (add oils to increase efficiency)

Use clothesline

Use "no heat" drying settings

Mist your clothing with dilute essential oils to freshen them or to hang them to dry

Add Essential oils to wash water to decrease need for warm water

Add Essential oils to Borax or baking soda, stir, and let sit for 5 minutes then add to wash

2. **Save Water**

   Decrease shower by 5 minutes

   Flush every other Flush

   Low flow shower head

   Faucet aerator

   Native landscaping

   Pour half full glass of water on the plants or in the dog dish not down the drain

   Chemical Free Bath & Shower Products rinse cleaner and quicker in shower to decrease time and will impact environment less

3. **Use Less Petrochemicals**

   Walk or Bike

   Telecommute

   Lobby for Mass Transit and safe bike and walk ways

   Pre-map the Route for your errands

   Car pool

   Once you are healthier and less chemical laden the easier it will be to walk and bike

4. **Eat Smart**

   Cut back on the meat in your meals

   Buy locally

   "Food Inc." Movie

   Use natural fruit and Veggie cleaner

   Compose

   Recycle containers

79

Use your own containers

Clean produce and food with essential oils

> Soak in a solution of sea salt and vinegar with several drops of *Citrus limon*, peel

> Fruits & Veggies will stay fresh longer and save lots of money

5. <u>Eliminate Plastic Especially Water Bottles</u>
Filter your own water

Fill your own bottles instead of delivery

Use reusable bottles like glass

Watch "The Story of Bottled Water" (YouTube)

Use a variety of Essential oils to Clean up Water and to add Flavor options while enhancing the systems natural detox or waste management systems.

6. <u>Think Before You buy</u>

Borrow instead of buying

Buy smart

Repurpose

Reuse

Buy used

Find something you already own and use it instead

Second hand / Gently Used

"The Story of Stuff" (YouTube)

Disinfect and Debug with Essential oils

Libraries

E-books

Co-op in your Neighborhood

Talk to your friends and neighbors about the Go Green Options

Buy in Bulk (saves packaging, Saves $)

Wear clothes that do not need to be dry-cleaned

High quality, long lasting, pay more less of a footprint

Test drive a friends' product and make sure it is what you want

Some of these oils will last for years with incredible benefits

One bottle of Purify blend will make 250 oz of cleaning product

Diffusing in the home will save hundreds on chemical based products

Invest in quality to get quality long-term use

7. <u>Keep Electronics Out of the Trash</u>

Use them as long as possible – There is a difference between need and want!

Donate or Recycle

Lobby for an electronics hazardous waste collection event

Use in art projects

Cut down on your EMF Pollution – Read from a book instead

Using Essential oils in the home will cut down on the harmful effects of the electronic devices in our home

8. **The more "Raw" the product the less taxing it is on the ecosystem**
    Donate or Recycle

    Eat and buy products that are eco-friendly and biodegradable

    Bring your own bags to the store

    Dispose of Waste responsibly

    Use products that did not go through processing

    Use Farmer Markets

    Rally for more local non processed products

    Rally for a co-op that uses minimal packaging and all biodegradable materials

    Support sustainable business

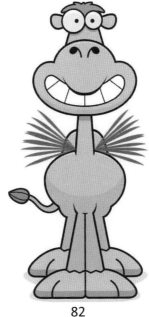

THE KEY - Buy less - Wrapped in less - That uses and leaves less

Ask how much energy, raw products and labor resources went into making this product

Be aware of:

1.   We are running out of natural resources

2.   Production = toxic synthetic products and more pollution

3.   Distribution = prices down, keep inventory moving and keep us rebuying

4.   Consumption = nation of consumers

        our primary way of our value is measured by stuff

        Only 1% in still in use after 6 months of what we buy

        99% becomes unwanted and discarded

5.   Disposal = not enough room we have a floating plastic island in the ocean!

        4.5#s of garbage produced per day per person

        Burning producing super toxins in incinerators = Dioxin

6.   Recycling helps

        It will never be enough

        70x as much garbage is produced to make the stuff

7.   We must create a new model that does not use the old consumer model.

9. Host Parties That Teach Awareness

Play the "It just might be TOXIN Game"

GAME

1. Go through labels and eliminate where you can

If a product label says   Caution – Warning - Danger -
ANYWHERE   It is a toxin!!

Make a contest out of who can find the most and what
to replace it with.

BE & USE GO GREEN ALTERNATIVES!!!

DO NOT GET TRAPPED BY MARKETING PLOYS THAT
ARE OVER PRICED NOVELTY GO GREEN TRAPS.

If you cannot pronounce it throw it out

2.   Research and present the latest findings

They have conclusive evidence that DEA can be
absorbed via skin and it is still in products. How long
before the other chemicals are found out too? It took
20 years for a label on tobacco.

How are they overwhelming our defenses?

Could there be any interactions or compounds formed
from interactions on our skin

3.   Apply the steps to Going Green to every product and item of stuff you have.

Ask can I recycle this?

Can I repurpose this?

Can I donate or sell this?

Can I buy this used?

How many resources will it take for me to own this?

Find Green companies and support them.

Many companies now take discarded items and repurpose them for 3rd world countries. Ask if maybe you could donate to those in need.

4.   Create a list of ideas to enhance this movement.

5.   Teach people simple green recipes such as the ones below.

Teach Bio-sustainability.

6.   Make and take new green recipes

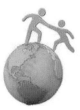

"We can't help everyone, but everyone can help someone."

- Ronald Reagan

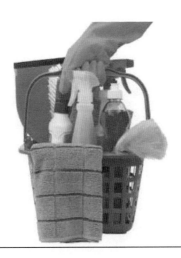

10. Make Your Own Cleaning Supplies With the essential Oil Advantage

Effective & Non-toxic & Simple

Saves $$, time, packaging and waste

Improves air Quality

E. <u>Backyard Go Green Alternatives:</u>

Composting

Nature's way of recycling

Reduces waste

Great for organic plants, lawns and gardens

Conserves resources

Conserves water

Conserves energy and fuel

Saves you money

Can be very educational

<u>Spray for Deodorizing Yard</u>

Poop Smell B'Gone

12 ounces distilled water

Pinch baking soda

½ tsp vodka or witch hazel

12 drops Purify blend (For recipe go to www.safe4animals.com)

4 drops *Pelargonium graveolens,* flower

Mist as needed

Spray for Insecticides

Anti-Parasitic Spray

10 drops *Cedrus atlantica* bark   3 ounces distilled water

10 drops *Rosmarinus officinalis* leaf   1 ounce Apple Cider Vinegar

10 drops *Cymbopogon nardus*

10 drops *Citrus limon* peel

Combine in spray bottle and apply via misting every 72 hours for heavy coverage to yard (during outdoor events up to 3 times a day) or monthly spray around the perimeter of the home and on door jams to keep pests outdoors

Spray for Fertilizers

Organic Beauty for lawn & household plants

¼ cup castor oil   1 gallon distilled water

¼ cup apple cider vinegar   40 drops *Ocimum basilicum* leaf

20 drops of *Boswellia carterii* resin   40 drops of *Cymbopogon flexuosus* leaf

Spray weekly to yard and household plants as needed . Every 2-4 weeks after sunset.

Fertilizing the Garden Plants

Add 6 drops of chosen essential oil to 2 gallons of water and mist plants after sunset

Ocimum basilicum, leaf	Grass, Roses, Potatoes, Tomatoes, Asparagus, Green beans, Broccoli
Mentha piperita, leaf	Cabbage
Salvia officinalis	Carrots, Cauliflower, Cucumbers
Pelargonium graveolen, flower	Peas, Peppers
Lavendula angustifolia	Fruit and Grapes
Boswellia carterii, resin & *Cymbopogon flexuosus,* leaf	Encourage plant growth

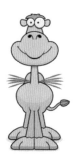

Garden Pesky Pests Potion

8 drops of essential oil to 1 gallon of water & 1 ounce vodka or witch hazel

Mist plants down after sunset weekly or soak fabric strips or string for 5 minutes in product and hang around the plants. Shake well before each use.

Rosmarinus officinalis, leaf	Caterpillers, cats
Mentha piperita, leaf	Mice, rats, spiders, aphids, ants, beetles, fleas, moths, plant lice
Pogostemon cablin	Snails, weevils, wooly aphids
Lavandula angustifolia & *Cymbopogon flexuosus,* leaf	Chiggers, mosquitoes, ticks
Thymus vulgaris, leaf	Chiggers, ticks, roaches
Syzygium aromaticum , flower bud	Flying insects
Thymus vulgaris, leaf & Cutworm *Salvia officinalis*, leaf	
Piper nigrum, fruit	Dogs, herbivores
Cedrus atlantica, bark & *Hyssop officinalis* & *Pinus sylvestris*	Slugs and snails -place in ring around plant
Melaleuca alternifolia & Cymbopogon nardus	Fungus
Pogostemon cablin & *Melaleuca quinquenervia*	Mildew and Fungus

Attract Pollinators Please

8 drops of essential oil to 1 gallon of water & mist plants down after sunset weekly. Shake well before each use.

Coriandrum sativum, seed or Citrus aurantium, flower	Bees
Achillea millefolium, leaves/flowers or Foeniculum vulgare, seed or Salvia officinalis, leaf	Butterflies

Suppress Fungus Spray

2 Tbsp Neem oil	1 cup distilled water
5 drops Rosmarinus officinalis, leaf	3 drops Cinnamomum verum, bark
2 drops *Origanum vulgare*, leaf/stem	3 drops *Thymus vulgaris*, leaf
6 drops *Mentha piperita*, leaf	3 drops *Syzygium aromaticum*, flower bud

Mix all together & spray after sunset weekly. Shake well before each use.

Mildew and Fungus Protection

10 drops *Pogostemon cablin*

10 drops *Melaleuca quinquenervia*

1 gallon Water

½ tsp Castile soap

Mix well together and mist after sunset monthly or more if needed. Shake well before each use.

Slip Sliders Slug & Snail Away

10 drops *Cedrus atlantica,* bark

10 drops *Hyssop officinalis*

10 drops *Pinus sylvestris*

16 ounces of water

1 tsp apple cider vinegar

Combine all ingredients, shake well before each use. Place in a ring around the plant on the ground.

USE reusable Clean

New Sprayers

Essential oils
dissolve plastics
so consider glass
or stainless steel.

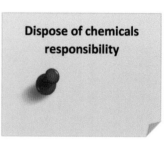

**Dispose of chemicals
responsibility**

A 5 Gallon Internal Tank Solvent Sprayer is a chemical spray

applicator with an all stainless steel cart assembly that is

suitable for handling many higher-flash-point solvents.

Connect compressed air to pressurize the 316L stainless steel

ASME rated tank and project ready-to-use solution through the

hose, wand and fan pattern spray nozzle.

You will get 7-15 minutes of spray time per canister.

F: Garage Go Green Alternatives

Understand hazardous waste.

Hazardous waste cannot be disposed of like normal trash in landfills. Instead it must be disposed of through the proper networks to prevent human and environmental harm.

Look at the characteristics of hazardous waste:

Ignitability means that the waste can easily catch on fire. It is considered flammable if the flash point is less than 140 degrees Fahrenheit.

Corrosive wastes are acids/bases that are capable of corroding metal containers.

Reactive wastes are unstable under normal conditions. They can cause explosions, toxic fumes, gases or vapors when heated.

Toxic types of wastes are potentially fatal or harmful when absorbed or ingested. They can pollute groundwater if not disposed of properly.

Be responsible with your waste.

Responsibility in disposing these types of wastes isn't just for your carbon footprint. Many counties and states attach legal responsibility towards disposing hazardous waste.

Companies who don't adhere to the laws are subject to fines and other legal action.

Research your local laws.

Many counties across the U.S. have specific protocol for disposing hazardous waste. Each county can have different steps and regulations for disposing hazardous waste. The actual disposal of hazardous waste on the local level is enacted by the Environmental Protection Agency (EPA).

Essential Oils as Degreasers

Orange oil or any of the citrus oils make the best degreasers

Garage Grease

½ cup salt

½ cup washing soda

2 cups baking soda

Stir well

Add ¼ cup water to make a paste

Spread paste on grease and let it set 30 minutes

Then

Mix ¾ cup distilled white vinegar

10drops *thymus vulgaris*

10 drops *citrus limon*

10 drops *citrus sinensis*

Shake well

Spray over the paste

Wipe clean with damp cloth

Combat VOC's

Create ventilation

Remove carpet and low VOC paint

Potted Greenery

Eliminate scent-releasing products

Pots of water with essential oils in them around the house renew often

Spray all furniture, carpet, and walls with essential oils to decrease off gassing

Diffuse 2 times a day for 30 minutes with ventilation

Store chemicals elsewhere

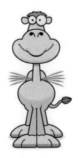

Diffuse in the Garage

Diffuse every 12 hours

1. Purify blend 10-20 drops

2. Combine 5 d *Eucalyptus radiata*, leaf

    5 d *Boswellia carterii*, resin

    5 d *Citrus limon,* peel

3. Combine 8 d *Abies balsamea*, Canada needle

    8 d *Commiphora myrrha*

    8 d *Citrus sinensis,* peel

4. Combine 6 d *Eucaluptus globulus*

    6 d *Cinnamomum camphora*

    6 d *Melaleuca quinquenervia*

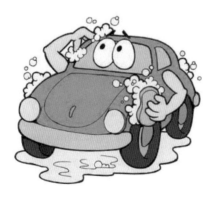

Go Green Car wash

Clear Musty Air

> 1 cup White Vinegar
> 4-6 drops essential oil(s) of choice
> 1 slice of bread

Fill a small bowl with vinegar and essential oils. Add a piece of bread on top of liquid and place inside the vehicle to absorb odors. Remove after 24 hours.

Easy Citrus Car Wash

> 1 gallon water
> 1/4 cup Castile Soap
> 10 drops *Citrus limon*, peel & *Citrus sinensis*, peel oil

Fill a bucket with the water and soap, stir until mixed and then add the essential oil and stir again. Using a soft cloth or sponge, wash the exterior of your car from top down, one section at a time. Rinse each area well with clean water before the soap has a chance to dry. Avoid using in direct sunlight.

Tough-to-Get Dirt

> 1 gallon Water
> 1/2 cup Lemon Juice
> 6 drops *Eucalyptus globulus* & *Mentha spicata* oil
> 1/4 cup Liquid Castile Soap
> 3 tablespoons Baking Soda

Mix water, lemon juice, essential oil(s), and soap in a bucket and stir in baking soda until blended. With a soft cloth or sponge, wash the exterior of your car from the top down, working in sections. Rinse each area well with clean water before the soap dries. Avoid using in direct sunlight.

Tire Wash

> 2 cups Baking Soda
> 1/2 cup Water
> 1/4 cup Liquid Castile Soap
> 2 cups Vinegar or Lemon Juice
> 5 drops *Citrus limon, Citrus sinensis*, &
>   *Citrus latifolia* oil

Combine baking soda, water, and soap in a bucket or other container. Add the vinegar and essential oil(s) and mix well. Apply with a brush to get in between the tire treads. Wash one tire at a time, rinsing each before moving on to the next. Avoid using in direct sunlight.

Lavender Leather Upholstery Cleaner

> 1/2 cup Mineral soap (safe4animals.com)
> 1 cup Hot Water
> 6 drops *Lavandula angustifolia* oil

Dissolve soap in hot water. Add essential oil and blend well. Apply formula with a soft brush, using gentle downward strokes. Wipe with a clean, damp cloth. Buff dry with a towel. Avoid using in direct sunlight. Follow with the Upholstery Conditioner (below)

Fragrant Leather Upholstery Conditioner

> 1/2 cup Olive Oil
> 1/4 cup Strong Rosemary Tea
> 1/4 cup Vinegar

Combine all ingredients in a plastic spray bottle and shake well before every use. Lightly spray onto upholstery and buff with a dry cloth. Avoid using in direct sunlight.

Carpet Upholstery Deodorizer

> 1/2 cup Baking Soda
> 10 drops *Lavandula angustifolia* oil
> (or oil of your choice)

Add oils to baking soda and mix well with a fork. Break up oil clumps to insure the oil is evenly distributed. Sprinkle liberally over your carpets and upholstery. Leave for a half hour. Vacuum off. When you vacuum your caret, move the vacuum very slowly, going with the grain of the carpet. Avoid using in direct sunlight.

Dashboard Restorer

> 1 cup Water
> 1/2 cup Mineral soap
> 10 drops *Cedrus atlantica*, bark oil

Combine all ingredients in a small plastic spray bottle and shake well. Spray onto dashboard and wipe clean with a soft cloth. Avoid using in direct sunlight.

Air Freshener Ideas

1. Wooden clothespin

   Soak in essential oil of choice(20 Minutes)

   Clip to air vent in the car to freshen air

   Recharge weekly

2. Cut a bar of essential oil infused soap up into squares and place beneath seat for a slow release of fragrance.

   Place in small Mason jar with cheesecloth on the top to trap melted soap and to still allow release of the scent.

3.   Soak fabric strips or string in essential oil mix and hang or tie
        where desired

              Mix ¼ cup water

              1 Tbsp of vodka or witch hazel

              15 drops of essential oil of choice

Mat and Carpet Cleaner

              1/2 gallon Hot Water
              1/2 cup Liquid Castile Soap
              12 drops *Gaultheria procumbens*, leaf &
              Mentha piperita, leaf oil

Combine all ingredients in a bucket or pail. Stir thoroughly to mix.

Vacuum loose dirt from carpeting and mats. Remove mats from the car
and clean by dipping a brush into the cleaning solution and rubbing
into the carpet fibers. Rinse the mats with a hose and allow them to
dry in the sun.

Clean the carpeting on the floor of the car by dipping brush into the
cleaning solution and rubbing into the carpet. Wipe with a dry towel.
Vacuum again when completely dry. Avoid using in direct sunlight.

One Stop Shopping   -- Anti-Microbial Blend Pre-Made Product Line

        Use diluted Anti-microbial Cleaner Blend (safe4animals.com)

        Use to clean and freshen everything

        Cut small pieces from the bar soap and use as air fresheners

        Use hand soap to condition leather

G. City Neighborhood Walks, Parks and Hikes Go Green Alternatives

Act as own diffuser

Before you leave: Mist them down to protect them on their romp in the park they can act as their own diffuser and purify the air around them more. There is less likelihood bugs will jump on with the smell of oils. Afterward it will decrease the load of chemicals they picked upon their fur.

After the Romp: Mist them down then wipe them off. Research showed that reduces particulate matter on the fur by over 90%. At times Protective gear may be a good deterrent to picking up chemicals.

Spray for Disinfection

Coat of Armor Spray on Protection

16 ounces distilled water

1 ounce apple cider vinegar

16 drops Purify blend

5 drops *Cedrus atlantica.* bark

5 drops *Chameacyparis formosensis,* wood

Mist pet before going out on adventures. Mist every 2-3 hours to reset effect.

Wipe Down

90% of debris, chemicals and allergens can be removed just by wiping your pet down upon returning.

Cut up and repurpose old cotton or bamboo T-shirts into "Baby Wipe" sizes

Package into used containers free of chemical residue

Mix in Mason jar

> 16 ounces distilled water
>
> 4 ounces vodka or witch hazel
>
> 10 drops Purify blend
>
> 10 drops *Cymbopogon citratus* leaf
>
> 10 drops *Chameacyparis obtuse*

Mix liquid together

Saturate cotton t-shirts and store in tightly closed container

Retain remaining liquid in spray bottle to mist areas and/or wipe pet down with homemade wipes.

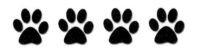

Foot Bath

Clean your pet's feet after returning from a romp in the park. They have collected a lot of visitors and there is no need for them to lick themselves clean and ingest them. Chemicals can be absorbed through the skin, inhaled and then ingested to create a triple whammy effect of intoxication.

Magic Toes

Have a sweater box or flat container prefilled with water

Add 1/4 cup of Pre-charged Epsom salts or sea salts per gallon of water & stir well

Allow pet to stand in water 1-5 minutes or at least walk through the water

Many of my clients will even have this set up at the doggie door with a towel on the other side so the pet washes their feet every time they use the doggie door.

Pre-charge the salts with essential oil of choice:

10 drops Purify blend

10 drops *Cymbopogon citratus,* leaf

10 drops *Chameacyparis obtuse*

10 drops *Pinus sylvestris*

10 drops *Citrus sinensis,* peel

Add 20-30 drops of selected above oils per cup of dry salts

Stir well into dry salts.

Let sit at least 5 minutes covered and sealed

Then disperse into the warm water

Detox bath

Let Bath Time be Detox Time

1 cup of Epsom salts or sea salt

15 drops of *Cymbopogon flexuous,* leaf

15 drops of *Citrus paradisi* ,rind

Stir into dry salt and let sit at least 5 minutes, cover and seal tightly

Immerse pre-charged salt into tub of water, disperse and dissolve

Allow pet to soak or ladle over pet for 5 minutes

Rinse pet very well, drain water

Add 1 cup of apple cider vinegar to new tub of water

Ladle over pet and allow to air dry

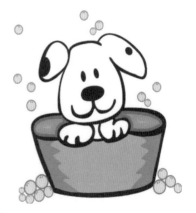

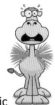

<u>OMG What was That They Ate Tonic</u>

OMG Tonic

From time to time our pets eat something along their journey. In many pets this shows up later in the form of anorexia, vomiting or diarrhea

To assist on the way to the vet or to be on the safe side use the following:

> 2 tsp coconut oil
>
> ½ tsp lemon juice
>
> ½ tsp apple cider vinegar
>
> 5 drops *Helichrysum italicum,* flower
>
> 5 drops *Copaifera officinalis* ,wood oil

Stir all ingredients together well

Give with a dropper or syringe into mouth.

¼ tsp per 10# body weight any time after an OMG ingestion incident

Still seek veterinary advice.

Add ¼ tsp baking soda to the mix and allow bubbles to settle to help if there is vomiting or acid reflux see **"First Aid for pets with Veterinary Medical Aromatherapy®" by Dr. Nancy**

Insect Repellent Spray

Biting Bug B Gone

16 ounces distilled water   1 ounce apple cider vinegar

1 ounce vodka or witch hazel

10 drops each of:

> *Cymbopogon nardus*
>
> *Lavandula angustifolia*
>
> *Citrus limon,* peel
>
> *Pelargonium graveolens,* flower
>
> *Nardostachys jatamansi*

Combine ingredients, shake well before each use, mist pet every 8 hours for protection

Purify Blend Repellent

16 ounces of distilled water   1 ounce apple cider vinegar

16 drops of Purify blend

Mix, shake well before each use and mist pet every 8 hours

www.safe4animals.com for easy pre made product options also

Heat Stroke ER Spray

4 drops *Lavandula angustifolia*

10 drops *Mentha piperita,* leaf

8 drops *Eucalyptus glabulus*

8 ounces distilled water

1 Tbsp vodka or witch hazel

Mix together, place in Mason jar

Store in refrigerator

Mist on pets feet, belly, and back after exposure to excessive heat

Still seek veterinary care

H. Kitchen Go Green Alternative

Dishwasher Detergent

1 cup Borax   1 cup Washing soda (Arm & Hammer)

10 drops of essential oil of choice that is safe for ingestion

Combine ingredients together

Use 1/8 cup per load
If hard water adjust by adding an extra ½ cup Washing soda or more as needed

Dishwasher Detergent #2

1 cup Baking Soda   10 drops *Citrus sinensis,* leaf
¼ cup citric acid   1 cup Borax
15 drops *Citrus lemon,* peel
Mix together. Add a sachet of white rice to container to absorb moisture.
Use 2 Tbsp per load

Glass Cleaner

Combine   ½ cup white vinegar
                 ½ cup distilled water
                 4 drops *Eucalyptus radiata* oil

Spray on glass or mirror wipe clean with newspaper
Test first on any glass or mirror with a plastic coating

Oven Cleaner

Make a paste of Baking soda 4 cups and Sea salt 1 cup using hot water
Coat oven, let sit 2 hours then wipe clean
Place a bowl of boiled water in oven infused with 10 drops of essential oils of choice
Close oven and let sit overnight to freshen oven odor

Do NOT use essential oils in hot oven.

All Purpose Cleaner

½ cup white vinegar

¼ cup baking soda

½ gallon water

10 drops *Citrus sinensis*, peel

Infuse baking soda with orange oil let it sit 5 minutes then add to vinegar and water mixture.

Store in Mason jars or used glass jars free of chemical residue

All Purpose Cleaner #2

2 tsp baking soda

Infuse with 8 drops of essential oil of choice

Add 1 2/3 cup water

Mix well, shake before each use, spray and wipe clean.

Softer Scrub

¾ cup baking soda

¼ cup castile soap

2 Tbsp water

5 drops each *Gaultheria procumbens*, leaf & *Mentha piperita*, leaf oil

Mix to form a paste
Store in covered container

Degreaser Cleaner for Surfaces

4 ounces baking soda

2 ounces THHC Pre made cleaner (safe4animals.com)

Form a paste

Add 25 drops of *Citrus sinensis*, peel oil to paste mix together

Wet surface with water

Place paste on sponge and scrub

Wipe away with damp cloth

Degreaser Spray for Surfaces

2 cups warm water

1 Tbsp baking soda

20 drops *Citrus limon*, peel oil

Mix together, shake well before each use, spray on grease and wipe clean with damp cloth.

Dish Soap

Premade THHC Products are available (safe4animals.com)

Cut the Grease Dish Soap

2 cups warm water

2 Tbsp baking soda

¼ cup castile soap

¼ cup lemon juice

40 drops each of *citrus limon*, peel & *citrus sinensis*, leaf & *citrus sinensis*, peel

Mix well, shake gently before use, store in glass well sealed

Kitchen Fresheners

1.   Many ideas are spread throughout this book.

2.   Simmer ½ cup vinegar, ½ cup water and 10 drops of choice:

Cymbopogon citratus, leaf   *Chamaecyparis obtuse*

Citrus sinensis, peel   *Chamaecyparis formosensis*, wo

Pinus sylvestris   *Citrus limon eureka* var. *formosensis* peel

On the stove while you are cooking to freshen cooking odors.

3.   Place coffee grounds in containers infused with essential oils like:

Syzygium aromaticum, flower bud

Myristica fragrans

Cinnamomum verum, bark

Elettaria cardamomum, fruit/seed

Zingiber officinale, root

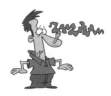

4.   Grind citrus rinds especially lemon in the garbage disposal to freshen add 2 drops of companion essential oil to enhance.

5.   To freshen food storage containers soak overnight in 4 parts warm water to 1 part baking soda and 1 part white vinegar add 10 drops of essential oil of choice to enhance.

6.   Use diffusers throughout your home.

Meat Disinfection/Tenderizer

2 cups water

3 Tbsp white vinegar

1/8th tsp baking soda

1 Tbsp olive oil

10 drops each *Piper nigrum*, fruit &

Citrus limon eureka var. *formosensis*, peel &

Citrus paradisi, rind

Allow meat to marinate for 30 minutes discard liquid then store in appropriate container in the refrigerator. The meat will be more tender and keep days longer in the refrigerator.

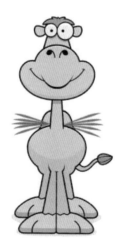

Fruit and Veggie Wash

In a sink full of water place 10-20 drops of Purify blend, stir well

Place all fruit and veggies to be washed into water, let sit 5 minutes then rinse

or

Use THHC pre made wash as an alternative

or

8 ounce of water add 8 drops of Purify blend or Citrus blend

Mix well and mist onto produce to be wiped clean

Or

2 cups of water
 1/4 cup baking soda
2 cups white vinegar
3 drops *Citrus limon*, peel
Place produce in sink
Sprinkle with baking soda
Add mixture of water oil and vinegar
Mix produce with hands and let soak for 30 minutes

Or

6 ounces white vinegar 6 ounces water
15 drops *Citrus limon*, peel
Combine in spray bottle and mist all produce as needed.

> *Citrus limon*, peel has d-limonene, up to 72%, making it perfect for dissolving synthetics such as the coating commonly used on fruits and vegetables.

114

Food Preservation with Essential Oils

Essential oils not only can remove the petrochemical laden film from produce and meats they will also serve to increase their freshness. Essential oils have been studies and used in the food industry for years as natural preservatives.

After washing produce thoroughly in essential oils mist them sown with a spry of oils then put into containers for proper storage.

Take a used cotton t-shirt strip and soak it in essential oil cleaner place on bottom of storage container then layer your cut and prepared produce on top. They will stay fresh sometimes up to two weeks.

For fresh herbs take a paper towel or cheesecloth mist with essential oil spray and loosely wrap herbs in toweling and place in crisper the herbs will stay fresh for days.

Your food will taste fresher and have more flavors now that the chemicals are gone.

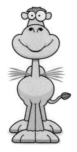

I. <u>Bathroom Go Green Alternatives:</u>

<u>Bathroom Surface Cleaner</u>

6 oz distilled water

6 oz white vinegar

10 drops *Citrus limon*, peel

12 drops *Lavandula angustifolia*

Mix together in 12 ounce spray bottle. Shake well before each use. Use on all surfaces spray on and wipe clean with a clean soft cloth like a used cotton T-shirt.

<u>Grub Scrub</u>

½ cup baking soda

5 drops *Citrus limon*, peel

1 capful THHC

3 drops Anti-microbial

essential oil blend

Combine ingredients to make a paste

Clean with a soft brush or clean soft cloth.

Rinse with water and damp cloth

Finish with dry soft cloth

Intended to use all product at once

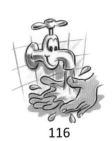

Foaming Hand Soap Ideas

2 Tbsp Liquid Castile soap unscented or Nature's rich soap

1 cup water

Essential oil formulation of choice. Use foaming soap dispenser.

Bathroom combination:

10 drops each of *Myrtus communis* & *Citrus sinensis*, peel

or

5 drops each of *Myrtus communis, Lavandula angustifolia* & *Cedrus atlantica*, bark

Kitchen combination:

5 drops each of *Lavandula angustifolia, Citrus limon*, peel

& *Rosmarinus officinalis*, leaf

General use:

THHC foaming hand soap **(safe4animals.com)**

Drain Cleaner

Place ¼ cup baking soda into drain

Then add 5 drops of *Citrus limon*, peel oil

Follow with ½ cup white vinegar

Close drain tightly until fizzing stops

Flush with 4-6 cups of boiling water

Use caution with plastic pipes.

Mildew and Mold Removers

    2 Tbsp lemon juice

    ½ cup white vinegar

Combine

Infuse 1 Tbsp sea salt with

10 drops *Pelargonium graveolens*, flower

Stir well, let sit for 5 minutes then

Disperse into lemon juice and vinegar.

Rub onto surfaces and wipe clean with a damp cloth.

Bathroom Mold Bubble Cleaner

    ¼ cup Hydrogen peroxide 3%

    ½ cup water

    combine into spray bottle

    In a separate spray bottle combine:

    4 ounces of water

    8 drops each of the following essential oils

    Cymbopogon citratus,leaf

    Pelargonium graveolens, flower

    Melaleuca quinquenervia

    Mist area first with essential oil spray

    Then mist over with the peroxide spray

    Let sit 1 hour then wipe clean with a damp cloth

Deodorizers

Air Freshener Ideas

1.   Live household plants

2.   Dishes with ½ cup baking soda, 2 Tbsp fresh lemon juice,

     5 drops each oil:
     Citrus limon, peel &
     Citrus sinensis, leaf &
     Citrus limon eureka var. *formosensis*, peel
              Or
     Citrus essential oil blend

3.   Diffusers

        No limits enjoy.

**Home Halitosis
Alternatives**

**Everyone's home can
get a little stale from
time to time.**

1. Make a pomander. Stud an orange with whole cloves and cure it in the oven on low heat for about an hour – or place it in a paper bag somewhere cool and dry for about six weeks. Hang it with a ribbon or set in a pretty bowl to sweetly scent the area. Reanimate using *Citrus sinensis*, peel oil 2 times a week.

2. Open the windows. Every house can benefit from a good airing out. On a day with good air quality and a slight breeze, open your windows for a few hours. Open windows on all sides of the house to create a cross breeze that gets air moving.

3. Simmer spices. You can simmer spices such as whole cinnamon, cloves, and nutmeg on the stovetop or in a simmering pot.

4. Odor absorbers: Use a neutral odor absorbent such as a box of baking soda in a stinky area, or sprinkle especially smelly spots (such as the garbage can) with a little vinegar and baking soda.

5. Vinegar can remove odors from surfaces when you spray a little on and wipe it up.

6. Create your own potpourri from bulk herbs, flowers, and spices and leave a little in a bowl.

7. Use essential oils. Never use heat to distribute an oil it can be toxic.

8. Put a little citrus peel down the garbage disposal and turn ion to de-stink your drain.

9. Eliminate cooking odors by placing a shallow bowl of vinegar nearest the scent.

10. Soak cotton ball in vanilla or any essential oil and place it in a bowl where you want your home to smell better.

Disinfectant Spray

2 tsp borax

4 Tbsp white vinegar

3 cups hot water

Combine

Add ¼ tsp liquid castile soap

10 drops of essential oil of choice

Purify blend

Anti- microbial blend:

Citrus blend

Evergreen blend

Citrus limon, peel

Eucalyptus globulus

Chamaecyparis obtusa

Citrus limon eureka var. *formosensis*, peel

Satureja Montana

Melaleuca alternifolia

Cymbopogon martini, leaves

Cinnamomum camphora

Toilet Bowl Cleaner

¾ cup borax

1 cup white vinegar

     10 drops Pinus sylvestris

     10 drops Eucalyptus globulus essential oils

Combine ingredients into container

Swish toilet bowl to wet thoroughly

Dump ingredients inside bowl and distribute over bowl

Let sit overnight

Scrub and flush away

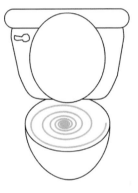

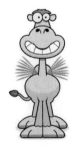

Replacing Personal Care item

50% of our personal care items are known carcinogens. They contain items like DEA – Diethanolamine, Propylene glycol or propanediol, or SLS. Many of these items have been grandfathered in by the FDA from as late as 1938. They are known to be absorbed via the skin and cause damage and yet are in items like shampoo, deodorants cosmetics, lotions, toothpaste, baby wipes and some pet foods.

Our pets often lick us with our creams and lotions. They may lick the shower after all the products were used. Many grooming products are of similar quality. Go to my website www.safe4animals.com for lots of replacement ideas.

Owie sprays and ointments - see" **First Aid with Veterinary Medical Aromatherapy® " www.safe4animals.com**

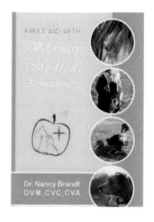

J. Bedroom Go Green Alternatives

Dry Cleaner Detox

Remove your items outdoors out of the bags

Hang outdoors and mist down with essential oil blends

Hang for 1 hour to air out and dissipate the chemicals

Avoid clothing that has to be dry cleaned if possible

Spritzers can be many essential oils add 5 drops to each ounce of water to assist in dissipation of dry cleaning chemicals.

Purify blend

Anti-microbial blend

Citrus blend

Evergreen blend

Citrus limon, peel

Eucalyptus globulus

Chamaecyparis obtusa

Citrus limon eureka var. *formosensis*, peel

Satureja Montana

Melaleuca alternifolia

Cymbopogon martini, leaves

Cinnamomum camphora

Chlorinated tris is still allowed in China in all bedding.
Let bedding material out gas in the warm sun for 24
hours before bringing it indoors. Buy organic wool.
Ask is it tested for VOC's?
Spray nightly with essential oils.

Bedding Deodorizer Dog

16 ounces of distilled water

10 drops Purify blend

10 drops Citrus sinensis, peel

Combine and shake well before each use. Mist pet bedding up to every 12 hours

Bedding Deodorizer Cat

16 ounces distilled water

pinch of baking soda

5 drops of Purify blend

3 drops of *Pelargonium graveolens,* flower

Combine and shake well before each use. Mist pet bedding up to every 24 hours

Pet Deodorizer

16 ounces distilled water

¼ tsp baking soda

20 drops Essential oils of choice

Purify blend is best

Shake before each use, mist pet as needed

Bedding Cleaner

4 ounces distilled water 2 ounces THHC

5 drops *Lavandula angustifolia*   15 drops Purify blend

5 drops *Melaleuca altnerafolia*

Combine ingredients into spray bottle, shake well, spray full contents over mattress , pillows and comforter and allow to air dry.

Air Fresheners

Spritzer sprays as above or other ideas mentioned throughout this book

Diffuse at night for a deeper sleep and easier breathing

Put cotton balls with several drops of essential oils on them inside your pillowcase.

Leave bowls of water in place and add oils to them each night.

Leave a dish with baking soda and lemon juice with oil as above.

Keep all essential oils out of reach of pets and kids.

Visit www.safe4animals.com for many diffuser recipes like Dreaming and Purify blend.

K. Laundry/Utility Room Go Green Alternatives

Go Green Kitty Box Ideas Disposable

Repurpose containers that will be going into the landfill as kitty boxes. You can clean with products in this book, fill with biodegradable materials and then throw the entire thing away after the kitty is done with it.

Urine combining either with the cleaners, litter and/or plastic of many cat boxes turn off the cat from using the box and can even form a lethal ammonium chlorine gas.

No Odor Kitty Box Deodorizer

4 cups baking soda

25 drops of Purify Blend

Stir well, let sit 5-19 minutes then store in tight container

Sprinkle 1 Tbsp in the bottom of the box with each change

Kitty Box Cleaner

6 ounces distilled water

3 drops Purify blend

Combine, Shake well before each use, Mist over rinsed out box for disinfection

Fabric Softener Alternative

12 ounces distilled water

12 ounces White vinegar

½ tsp Nature's rich soap or THHC (safe4animals.com)

10 drops *Rosmarinus officinalis*, leaf

10 drops *Eucalyptus globulus*

10 drops *Citrus sinensis*, peel

Combine together, store in glass container sealed

Use 1Tbsp per load

Fabric Sheet Alternative

Wool Dryer Balls

6 per load

Add 4-8 drops of your favorite essential oils to one ball per load

They save money on drying time too!!

Liquid Laundry Detergent

What you will need:

Medium size saucepan

Measuring cups

Long handle wooden spoon

5 gallon bucket with cover

Ingredients

4 cups hot tap water	5 capfuls THHC
1 cup Arm and Hammer super washing soda	5Tbsp Mrs. Stewarts Bluing Agent
½ cup Borax	2 cups baking soda
1 bar grated Dr. Bronner's pure castile soap	

Directions

Grate soap into small pieces and set aside. Pour 4 cups hot tap water Into saucepan and add soap, stirring continually over low heat until Soap is melted and dissolved. DO NOT BOIL. Fill bucket half full of hot tap water and add melted soap, washing soda, baking soda, Borax, and THHC. Stir well until all powder is dissolved. Fill 5 gallon bucket to just below the top. Stir, cover and let sit overnight to thicken. Add bluing agent. Option: once thickened, mix with blender. Fill an empty liquid laundry detergent bottle half full with soap and fill the rest with tap water.
 * Non-HE Machines: 5/8 cup per load (approx. 180 loads)
 *HE Machines: ¼ cup per load (approx.. 640 loads)

Bleach Alternative

1 ½ cups hydrogen peroxide 3%

½ cup Fresh Lemon Juice

10 drops *Citrus limon*, peel

1 gallon water

Combine all ingredients, store in glass container, sealed well

Use ½ cup per load of laundry

Insect Repellent

2 ounces distilled water

15 drops *Bursera graveolens*, wood

15 drops *Lavandula angustifolia*

15 drops *Rosmarinus officinalis*, leaf

1 Tbsp THHC www.safe4animals.com

Mix together

Shake well before each use

Spray generously along all baseboards and doorways

Safe on all pets except cats, use Cat insect spray instead.

Cat Insect Deterrent Spray

2 ounces distilled water

2 drops Purify blend

2 drops *Bursera graveolens*, wood

2 drops THHC www.safe4animals.com

Mix together

Shake gently before each use

Spray along baseboards and doorways

Bug B Gone

16 ounces distilled water   1 ounce apple cider vinegar

1 ounce vodka or witch hazel

10 drops each of:

> *Cymbopogon nardus*
>
> *Lavandula angustifolia*
>
> *Citrus limon,* peel
>
> *Pelargonium graveolens,* flower
>
> *Nardostachys jatamansi*

Combine ingredients, shake well before each use, mist pet every 8 hours for protection

L. Living Room Go Green Alternatives

Carpet Deodorizer

½ cup baking soda

½ cup corn starch

40 drops Essential oil of choice

> EPA says there is 7x more pollution in air inside home than outside the home
>
> 100x more than acceptable levels due to cleaners alone

Combine ingredients

Stir well, let sit 5 minutes

Sprinkle on carpet and let sit 1-6 hours

Then vacuum in all directions

Carpet Stains:

Freshen and lift the Carpet stains and odors

½ cup white vinegar

½ cup water

10 drops *Cymbopogon citratus*, leaf

Combine into spray bottle

Mist on carpet and brush out to freshen and lift carpet

Heavy Duty Stain Lifter

½ cup sea salt

½ cup borax

½ cup white vinegar

15 drops *Citrus limon*, peel

Make into a past, rub into carpet

Let sit for 2-4 hours

Rub with a brush and then vacuum.

Fresh Grease Stain

Sprinkle with corn starch

Wait 30 minutes

Vacuum

Follow with Freshen and Lift formula

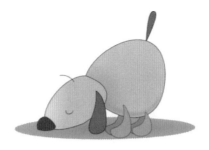

Freshen Up & Odor Control Ideas

Carpet

2 cups baking soda   36 drops of essential oils

Combine, stir well, let sit 5 minutes then sprinkle over entire carpet
Let sit 30 minutes or more then vacuum

Wood

Rub lemon wedge in and buff out

Electronics

1 cup white vinegar   ¼ cup baking soda
24 drops of essential oils of choice

Combine, shake well before use, wipe down all electronics

and allow to dry.

Buff to remove residue with soft recycled T-shirt

Freshen Furniture

Dusting Spray

1 cup white vinegar

½ tsp olive oil

3 cups water

15 drops Citrus sinensis, peel

15 drops Citrus limon,peel

Combine all ingredients into spray bottle

Shake well before each use

Mist and wipe clean

Furniture Polish

½ tsp olive oil

¼ cup white vinegar

½ tsp fresh lemon juice

10 drops *Pogostemon cablin*

10 drops *Vetiveria zizanoides,* root

Combine all ingredients, mix well, store in glass jar sealed well.

Dab a small amount on and spread out ward, then buff off. A little bit will go along way.

Sweet Mother of Wood Polish

8 oz sweet almond oil

4 capfuls of THHC

12 drops of *Citrus sinensis*, peel

Add all ingredients to spray bottle and shake well before each use.

Spray onto wood surface and wipe clean with a soft cloth.

M. <u>Office/Den Go Green Alternatives</u>

<u>EMF Diffusion Recipes</u>

1.   Combine 2 cups of water 1 tsp baking soda
      16 drops Purify blend
      Spray room down every 12 hours

2.   Place a diffuser in the room and diffuse Purify blend 2-3 times a
      day

3.   Place bowels of equal parts baking soda and pink Himalayan
      salt in the four corners of the room. Drop 5 drops of Purify
      blend in each bowl every morning.

EMF Spray

1 cup white vinegar	¼ cup baking soda
24 drops of essential oils of choice	Purify blend best choice

Combine, shake well before use, wipe down all electronics and
allow to dry. This will bubble, allow bubbles to settle.
Buff to remove residue with soft recycled T-shirt

EMF Absorbers

USB diffusers for essential oils

EMF disruptors

Do you know the amount of time
each American spends in front
of a EMF producing device?

Phone, TV, computer WiFi microwave According to
www.statista.com in 2014 it was 11 + hours a day.
That is A LOT of EMF pollution!!

N. Grooming Go Green alternatives
BATHS

Therapeutic Bath Soak

What you will NEED:

Oversized bowl for mixing	funnel
Wired whisk	3 glass bottles
Measuring cups	

INGREDIENTS

4 cups dry milk powder	2 cups dead sea salt (course or fine)
2 cups corn starch	1 cup Epsom salt
2 cups baking soda	24-48 drops of your favorite Biologically Active© Essential Oil.

DIRECTIONS – mix together dry ingredients with wire whisk until well blended. Pour into selected bottles 2/3 full. Add 8-16 drops your of your favorite Biologically Active© Essential Oil per bottle, shake until well blended (adding more Biologically Active© Essential Oil if desired). Fill bottle completely with dry ingredients and one more drop of EO to the top.

Use ½ a cup or more if desired per warm bath.

Will bubble with jetted tub.

Anti- Itch Bath Soak

2 cups dry goat milk powder	¼ c Dead Sea Salt (fine)
1 cup corn starch	3 Tbsp Oatmeal pulverized (coffee grinder)
1 cup Baking soda	15-30 drops essential oil

Directions:

Mix together all ingredients with wire whisk until well blended. Fill container of choice. Use ¼-1/2 cup per sink full of water for soak.

Suggested essential oils:

Pelargonium graveolens, flower, *Lavandula angustifolia*, *Lippia alba*, leaf/steam, or *Pogostemon cablin*

Anti-Parasitic Bath Soak

10 drops *Cedrus atlantica*, bark	3 ounces Apple Cider vinegar
10 drops *Rosmarinus officinalis*, leaf	1 ounce witch hazel or vodka
10 drops *Cymbopogon nardus*	¼ tsp baking soda
10 drops *Citrus limon*, peel	5 ounces Mineral soap

Combine in container. Disperse into tub. Soak old cotton T-shirts in water and wrap animal in cloth and ladel bath water over them for 10 minutes. Rinse them well.

After they air dry rub them down with Anti parasitic oil

Anti-Parasitic Oil Rub

¼ cup Sweet almond oil

¼ cup coconut oil

¼ cup jojoba oil

Combine oils.

Add 10 drops *Vetiveria zizanoides*, root

Add 10 drops *Copaifera officinalis,* wood

Add 10 drops *Leptospermum scoparium*, branch/leaf

Mix well, apply thin layer to every aspect of the fur and skin and allow to dry on pet.

Cat & Dog Tick/Flea Powder

4 cups Brewer's Yeast

10 drops each:

Cymbopogon nardus

Lavandula angustifolia

Citrus limon, peel

Pelargonium graveolens, flower

Nardostachys jatamansi

In an empty chemical free container, combine all ingredients, shake well

Rub into pets coat every other day

1 Tbsp per 10# body weight

No Odor Kitty Box Powder

4 cups Baking Soda

25 drops of Purify Blend

Stir well let sit 5-10 minutes then store in tight container and sprinkle 1 tbsp in the bottom of box with each change.

Kitty Box Cleaner

6 ounces distilled water

3 drops Purify blend

Mist over rinsed out box for disinfection

Dog Bedding Deodorizer

16 ounces of distilled water

10 drops Purify Blend

10 drops *Citrus limon*, peel oil

Mist pet bedding up to every 12 hours

Cat Bedding Deodorizer

16 ounces distilled water

Pinch of Baking Soda

5 drops Purify blend

3 drops *Pelargonium graveolens*, flower essential oil

Mist pet bedding up to every 24 hours

Pet Breath Deodorizer

5 drops *Mentha piperita*, leaf

2 drops Anti-Microbial blend

3 tsp of coconut oil

Mix well cover tight apply to gums once a day

Odor Control for Pets

16 ounces of distilled water

10 drops *Pelargonium graveolens*, flower

5 drops *Mentha spicata*

2 drops *Citrus limon*, peel

Mix together

Shake well before each use

Mist pet daily while covering their eyes

142

Pest Control Powder

1 cup diatameceous earth

5 drops *Cedrus atlantica*, bark

5 drops *Mentha piperita*, leaf

5 drops *Cinnamomum verum*, bark

Stir together and let sit 5-10 minutes

Sprinkle through-out the entire home under furniture especially

Insect Deterrent Spray

2 ounces distilled water

15 drops *Bursera graveolens*

15 drops *Lavandula angustifolia*

15 drops *Rosmarinus officinalis*, leaf

1 Tbsp THHC www.safe4animals.com

Mix together

Shake well before each use

Spray generously along all baseboards and door ways

Safe on all pets except cats use cat insect spray instead

Cat Insect Deterrent Spray

2 ounces distilled water

2 drops purify blend

2 drops *Bursera graveolens*

2 drops nature's rich soap www.safe4animals.com

Mix together

Shake gently before each use

Spray along base boards and door ways

Ear Cleaner !!

Use on external ear do not use in canal!!

1 ounce apple cider vinegar

1 ounce coconut oil

1 ounce distilled water

1 drop *Hyssop officinalis*

1 drop *Copaifera officinalis*, wood

1 drop *Lavandula angustifolia*

1 drop *Melaleuca alternafolia*

Mix together place 4 drops on cotton ball and place into canal but can still remove easily let sit there 10-15 minutes

Rub 2-3 drops around base of ear also

Pet Shampoo

3 ounces Liquid Castile Soap Unscented or nature's rich soap www.safe4animals.com

3 ounces distilled water

1 tsp sunflower oil, organic

2 drops *Citrus limon*, peel oil

2 drops *Pelargonium graveolens*, flower

2 drops *Lavandula angustifolia*

Combine all except soap shake well then add soap

Use ½ tsp per 20# rinse repeat

Detangler

1 tbsp Mineral Soap

1tsp Coconut oil

3 ounces distilled water

3 drops *Lavandula angustifolia*

2 drops *Pelargonium graveolens*, flower

1 drop *Cedrus atlantica*, bark

2 drops *Leptospermum scoparium*, branch/leaf

Shake well

Mist on to detangle

Consider premade products at safe4animals.com

Cleaning Products

Is the groomer using products that are both green friendly and will
keep bugs and diseases off your pet?

Manage Noise

Is the groomer managing noise pollution? Do they give breaks/ do they
have an area that is away from the noise? Do they use their inside
voice?

Manage emotions & Manage thoughts

Manage Boundaries / Restraint

How do they treat your pet? How do they treat each other? What
does the energy feel like? Does your pet want to go back or are they
running away?

Spa Treatments

Has your groomer been trained in Veterinary Medical Aromatherapy® and offer Spa treatments for your pets that are both safe and effective? Never let your groomer do a procedure they have not been trained for. Never let your groomer use products on your pet that contribute to their toxic load.

O. <u>Food/Water Go Green alternatives:</u>

See Dr. Nancy's book "Evolutionary Feeding of Pets"

Visit www.safe4animals.com

<u>Fruit and Veggie Wash</u> see kitchen

<u>Cleaner for Surfaces</u>   see kitchen

<u>Cleaner for Bowls</u>   see kitchen

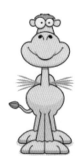

147

Bone Conditioning Soak

½ cup apple cider vinegar

2 drops of *Piper nigrum*, fruit

5 drops of *Citrus limon*, peel

5 drops of *Citrus latifolia*

2 drops of *Copaifera officinalis*, wood

Mix all contents together

Disperse into sink full of warm water to cover with bones to disinfect

Allow to soak for 5-10 minutes

Package to store

Meat will last longer and be safer for pets to eat raw or prepared

Meat Conditioning Soak

½ cup apple cider vinegar

5 drops of *Citrus limon*, peel

5 drops of *Citrus latifolia*

5 drops of *Cymbopogon flexuosus,* leaf

Mix all contents together

Disperse into sink full of warm water to cover with meat to disinfect

Allow soaking for 5-10 minutes

Package to store

Meat will last longer and be safer for pets to eat raw

Freshen That Water

Use ¼ tsp baking soda and add 1 drop of *Citrus limon*, peel

Stir and allow to sit for 5 minutes disperse into 1 gallon of water and give to pet as needed

Bowl Alternatives

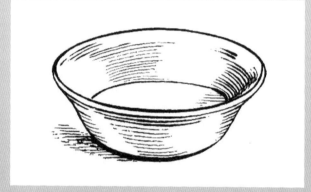

bamboo \ stainless steel \ glass

Repurpose what you already have. Best way to lessen footprint.

Eco friendly, biodegradable food containers come in many varieties—trays, bowls, plates and more. They're available in different sizes, with or without lids. They're also offered in natural and earth colors that make them stand out from other containers. Although they are made from plant fibers, they're extremely durable and safe for use in ovens and freezers. So if you're looking for the best food containers, eco-friendly food

P. Supplements Go Green Alternatives

See Dr. Nancy's book "Evolutionary Feeding of Pets"

Visit www.safe4animals.com

Essential oils as supplements and appropriate ways to give them

How to read labels

Food as alternatives

Food recipes as supplements

Q. Toy/Training Go Green Alternatives

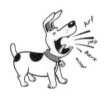

Find a trainer who talks your pet's language

Animal behaviorists can be educated in a variety of disciplines, including psychology biology, zoology or animal science. A professional applied animal behaviorist has demonstrated expertise in the principles of animal behavior, in the research methods of animal behavior, in the application of animal behavior principles to applied behavior problems and in the dissemination of knowledge about animal behavior through teaching and research.

Meat

Use small pieces of tasty clean meat to train. If you would not eat it (hotdog) do not give it to your pet.

Bones

Use raw meaty appropriately fed bones to supple the psychological needs of your pet. Be trained on safely feeding bones.

Freeze Dried

There are many products on the market that are freeze dried organ meats and animal parts. These are very convenient and so much better than a processed packaged product of no nutritive value. Organ meat is a great treat to help your pet's health also. Make sure the treats are appropriate size and shape so they will chew them not swallow whole

Engage the Mind

Be a big part of their life. Have a schedule they can count on. Commit. Pets are not a consumerized product that should be discarded when they are no longer fun. This is a lifetime commitment.

Look for alternative products or repurposed items to do pet oriented things

     Biodegradable poop bags

     Biodegradable pet wipes

     Bamboo training pads

     Make your own toys

R. <u>Veterinary Care Go Green Alternatives</u>

Does the Vet feel Western Medicine is our friend?

Does the Vet find ways to reduce, recycle and reuse?

Does the Vet find alternatives and offers them?

Is the Vet is trained in alternatives VMAA.VET or AHVMA.org?

Does the Vet utilizes detoxification programs?

Does the Vet teach chemical free living?

Ask about vaccine programs

Ask about feeding programs

Ask about wellness programs

Ask about training philosophies

Does it feel Zen and harmonious?

Does it smell good?

Is your pet relaxed there?

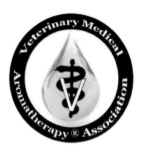

Find a Veterinary Medical Aromatherapy® trained Veterinarian at www.vmaa.vet

VMAA is the Veterinary Medical Aromatherapy Association

Founded in 2015 by Dr. Nancy Brandt the Pioneering Veterinarian in Veterinary Medical Aromatherapy®

The Tenants of Belief:

Promote Aromatherapy as a viable medical modality.

Provide standards of therapy that enhances the health and wellbeing of animals.

Create an alignment of all veterinary practitioners dedicated to establishing Veterinary Medical Aromatherapy®.

Set research and practice standards for the safe and effective use of aromatherapy in veterinary medicine.

Create an environment of non-partisan cooperation and sharing of information.

Provide exceptional training for professionals and the public.

CHAPTER SEVEN:

Why must we raise Chemical Free Pets?

PART 1: Sustainability

We must reduce our environmental impact. We must transform from consumerism to sustainability.

Get Motivated:

The Movie "Wall-E" should serve as an apt example of what the future holds if we do not change drastically our way of doing things to the planet.

Go Green:

Step back from marketing, step back from having our pets fulfill our needs to nurture and be nurtured. See our pets as part of the fragile ecosystem of the planet reminding us to return to our roots of cooperative living with nature. Our pets are serving to remind us to save this planet by any means necessary. That means Go Green, use nature again in a sustainable way and stop raping her resources and filling her up with unwanted previously wanted entertainment items.

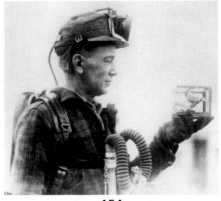

154

Use Nature as a Model:

Look to nature as an alternative way back to a sustainable world.

The circle of life.

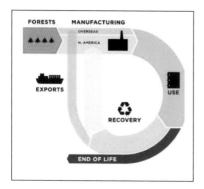
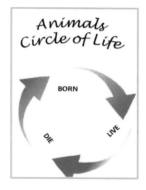

Educate Yourself:

"The Story of Stuff Project is changing the way we make, use and throw away stuff so that we can have a happier and healthier planet."

Build a Community:

Just like our pets are not disposable and turned in for the newer model we can also not turn in the Earth for a new model. Let's raise a chemical free Earth also. She's the only one we have.

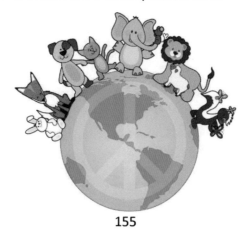

155

PART 2: Shopping list:

Lemons for fresh juice

Clean glass and mirrors
brighten your whites
disinfect
reduce sunspot,
wrinkles, pores
promotes detox functions
improves digestion and
immunity
sooth sore throats

Coconut oil

polish wood furniture
replace WD-40
remove Shower Scum
hair conditioner
gloss to lips and skin
deodorant
improve thyroid
decrease migraines
increase health of cell
membranes

Apple cider vinegar

repel fleas
clean microwave
deodorize
wash hair
adjust skin   pH
sooth sunburns
aftershave/waxing
treat skin infections
activate detox pathways
controls high blood pressure
controls yeast infections

White vinegar	polish silver
	clean windows
	remove hard water stains
	neutralize odors
	unclog drains
	tenderize meats
	eliminate odors
	keep produce fresh
	settles upset stomach
	soothe bee sting
	clarify hair
Baking soda	put out fires
	scrubbing power
	deodorant
	toothpaste
	relieve diaper rash /urine scald
	treat heartburn/acid reflux
	cooking assistant
Castile soap/mineral soap	dish soap
	cleaner
	body wash
	pet shampoo
	toothpaste
	moisture to skin
	decrease skin irritation
	and inflammation
Castor oil	discourage rodents
	lubricate items
	increase health of plants
	strengthen eyelashes
	relieve/ soften dry itchy skin
	laxative
	induce labor
	decrease menstrual cramps
	pulls toxins across and out of skin

PART 3: Biologically Active ®Essential Oils

1. Create an environment detrimental to pathogens
   - Anti-bacterial
   - Anti-fungal
   - Anti-viral
   - Anti-histamine
   - Anti-inflammatory
2. Shown to be effective in antibiotic resistant strains of bacteria

3. Bring negative ions, ozone and oxygen to the tissues
   - Regenerative nature

4. Create an environment of clear communication
   - Between all cells and all systems
   - Clean off receptor sites
   - Improve cell membrane function
   - Nutrition directly to the cell
   - Enhance neurotransmitters
   - Modulate enzyme activities
5. Create an environment detrimental to cancer cell growth
   - Erase or deprogram misinformation in cells

6. Emotional balancing and releasing stored memories
   - Links to the Instinctual Brain
   - Mend relationships
   - Erase negative energy
   - Mend abuse patterns
   - Discharge Emotional Toxicity
   - Modulate the human-animal bond and the created collective consciousness

7. Detoxify fat tissues
   Promotion of fat tissue drainage
   Clear impurities in Lipid matrix

8. Palliate and neutralize the harmful effects of
   Electromagnetic pollution
   Environmental pollution
   Air purification by both electrically charging
   the air and by disinfecting the air
   Clean impurities from the air

9. No negative chemical side effects

10. Economic way to be ecofriendly

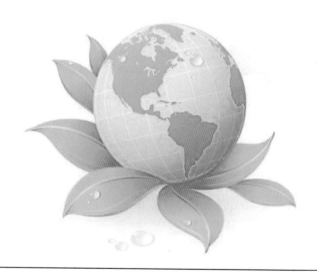

10 Best Essential oils for Green Cleaning

Citrus sinensis, peel
> Orange

Melaleuca alternifolia or *Melaleuca quinquenervia*
> Tea Tree

Rosmarinus officinalis, leaf
> Rosemary

Citrus limon, peel
> Lemon

Lavandula angustifolia
> Lavender

Eucalyptus globulus or *radiata*
> Eucalyptus

Mentha piperita, leaf
> Peppermint

Pinus sylvestris
> Pine

Thymus vulgaris, leaf
> Thyme

Cinnamomum verum, bark
> Cinnamomum

Biologically Active ®Essential Oils

www.safearomatherapy.com

This list surely looks better than the one we started with doesn't it??

PART 4: Solutions

Detoxification programs - see "Four Pillars of Health" book by

Dr. Nancy Brandt

1. We need to begin to:
   "Perform diagnostic testing for detection in the body and in the home"
2. Increase validity of energetic testing – applied kinesiology, pendulum, dousing etc.
3. Elimination of stored chemicals
4. Drink plenty of water
5. Improve lymphatic drainage
6. Utilize Homeopathic, Homotoxicology , herbal and essential oil protocols
7. Improve nutrition grain free diet in the carnivores
8. Increase digestion and intestinal care with Essential Oils
9. Utilize Essential Oils- see "Safe and Effective Veterinary Medical Aromatherapy" book by Dr. Nancy

Essential oils are able to release trapped toxins in the lipid matrix of the body and environment . Those are toxins that water would not flush away or aqueous supplements and drugs cannot impact. Essential oils are able to create significantly better lymphatic drainage. They are able to cross the blood brain barrier and clear the lipid matrix of the nervous system. The majority of toxins today are petrochemicals, such as plastics, that are lipid not aqueous in nature. Essential oils help clear the mesenchyme and remove trapped energetic signals. They are able to combat on the chemical level, electromagnetic level, emotional level and energetic level.

Without essential oils you are missing the trapped toxins that have built up in the fatty tissues of the body such as nervous, hormonal and lymphatic systems. Our top killers are lipid in nature – cholesterol, diabetes, obesity, infertility, lymphoma, mental health (autism, ADHD, depression) etc.

10. Environmental clean up

"To find out why you are sick simply recall what was new or different in your home, school or work area, or your diet, water or air immediately prior to the initial episode or any subsequent flare-up of your illness." (Rapp PG. 47) Any product you ingest, inhale or come in skin contact with needs to be evaluated. Environmental evaluations should include: dust, bacteria, molds, pet dandruff and hair, chemicals, pollen, toxic metals, electromagnetic exposures. (Rapp PG. 91)

11. Educational awareness

Host a Party – Train a Guardian – Save a pet

"One sensible answer appears not to be the need for another mind-altering overpriced drug, but recognition and elimination of the environmental causes of behavior and learning problems. (Rapp PG. 153) Common sense must be reinstated as a primary diagnostic tool. Utilizing the powers of deduction to become more aware of our impact on us by the environment we have created. Most industrial chemicals are on the market with no mandatory safety testing There is contamination in pet food, pet toys and other products for our companion animals have few standards that limit chemical contamination.

12. The Choice is Yours

PART 5: Obligations and Choices

1. **Our Contribution to the Toxic Overload**
   "Genetic changes can't explain the increases in certain health problems among pets. Scientists believe that chemical exposures play a role. (National Research Council 1991,) (Landrigan 2001)

2. **Our Responsibility to the Ecosystem**

   This is a call to action

   Begin with those you love – pets, children, friends and neighbors.

   Begin with the choices you make every hour of every day.

   Begin with opening up your eyes and seeing the effects around you.

   Begin by admitting you are at cause and your little bit does help.

                   (In the film Wall-e one robot saved earth)

   Demand the change by voting with your purchases

3. **Our choices for ourselves**
   "The bottom line is simple. If you personally resolve to clean up and stop polluting your nest, your food, your water, your air and your contacts, you and your loved ones will have a much better chance to become or remain well" I may add your thoughts and your emotional choices and also the electromagnetic impacts in the environment. Begin by using natural products with known therapeutic effects.

4. Essential impact of Therapeutic Grade Essential Oils:

a. Purity vs. adulterated - It makes no sense to use synthetically altered products in our attempt to clear the synthetic petrochemical impact when there are pure natural products which will alleviate the synthetic toxicity. Buy only Biologically Active®oils

b. Learn specific oils for specific pollutants
Pines and Citruses as cleaners and air fresheners are one example.

c. Environmental impact of essential oils. They are not contributing to the further contamination of the planet. How many pharmaceutical drugs are in our water supply now contributing to our environmentally impacted disease epidemic?

5. Conclusions:

There has been a drastic increase in such diseases as cancer and thyroid diseases, all of which have chemical links. According to Arlene Blum of the UC Berkeley chemistry department, "In lab animals, fire retardants were shown to cause hyperthyroidism" she went on to say, "chemicals are killing our pets and our people." (EWG 2008) By being closer to the ground our pets are exposed to higher concentrations of toxicity, and at the same time they are up to 20X less in body mass. They are our current day "Canary in the Coalmine". So what will you do to protect them now? What steps can you take to limit your exposure and contribution to the toxic wasteland? How will you protect the Canary and clean up the house?

The use of Therapeutic Grade Essential Oils on animals is both effective at alleviating toxic impacts upon them and is safe for the environment itself. Therapeutic Grade Essential Oils will not only clean up the mess of progress they will keep from contributing to the toxic dump, which our choices are creating. If they create better health and well-being, eliminating the toxic overload of an already polluted environment and they give back to the environment with a positive effect, why then are they not universally used???? The answer lies within your choices.

"The most important thing that you can do on this planet – elevate, transform and illuminate your own consciousness."

- Carlos Santana

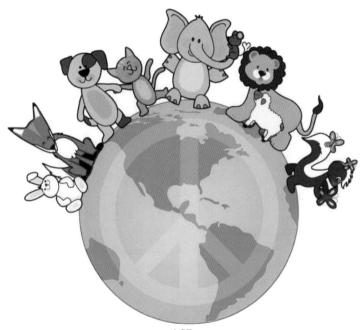

Resources and Notes:

FDA
"The Safe Shopper's Bible"
Warning Labels
EPA
OSHA
EWG
Blum, Arlene; "Did the State Kill my cat?" Los Angeles times, Oct 17,2008.
Dye JA, VenierM, ZhuL, Ward CR, Hites RA, Birnbaum LS, 2007. Elevated PBDE levels in pet cats; sentinels for humans? Environ Sci Technol 41(18): 6350-6
FDA CVM (U.S. Food and Drug Administration Center for Veterinary Me www.fda.gov/cvm/mission.htm [accessed April 2 2008].
FDA CVM (U.S. Food and Drug Administration Center for Veterinary Medicine). 2000b. Vision Statement. Available: www.fda.gov/cvm/visionstatement.htm [accessed April 2 2008].
Gunn-Moore D. 2005. Feline Endocrinopathies. Vet Clin North Am Small Journal of the American Veterinary Medical Association (JAVMA); "Research Finds High Concentrations of Chemicals in Pets" 2008.
Landrigan PJ. 2001. Children's environmental health. Lessons from the past and prospects for the future. Pediatr Clin North Am. 2001 48(5):
Naidenko, Olgg; Sutton, Rebbecca; Haulihan, Jane; "High Levels of Toxic Industrial Chemicals Contaminate Cats and Dogs" Environmental Working Group: April 2008 www.ewg.org/reports/pets
National Research Council (NRC). 1991. Animals as Sentinels of Environmental Health Hazards. Washington, DC: National Academies
Purdue University Department of Veterinary Pathobiology. 2000. Breed Health Surveys. Available http://www.vet.purdue.edu/epi/ [2008]
Rapp, Doris J., M.D.; "Our Toxic World" Environmental Medical Research Foundation Oct 2003; New York.
The Chemical Free Home by Melissa M. Poepping
Texas A&M Veterinary Medical Center. 2008. What is the incidence of cancer in our pets? Available: http://www.cvm.tamu.edu/oncology/faq/FAQ.html [2008].
Pictures of canaries in the mines providedto us by R C McDonald.
(Naidenko 2008) (JAVMA 2008)
www.natural-health-information-centre.com/sodium-lauryl-sulfate

www.angelfire.com/az/sthurston/alzheimers_and_aluminum_toxicity
www.cdc.gov/healthywater/other/agricultural/contamination.html
www.scientificamerican.com/article/tap-drinking-water-contaminants-
articles.mercola.com/sites/articles/archive/2005/01/19/whole-food-
supplements.aspx
empoweredsustenance.com/food-based-synthetic-supplements/
www.organicconsumers.org/news/vitamin-poisoning-are-we-
destroying-our-health-hi-potency-synthetic-vitamins
www.pcrm.org/research/resch/animalspsych
Environmentalhomecenter.com
Thegreenguide.com
saferchemicals.org/documents/backyard-bbq/
www.globalhealingcenter.com/natural-health/why-you-should-never-
microwave-your-food/
www.smithsonianmag.com/science-nature/five-reasons-why-you-
should-probably-stop-using-antibacterial-soap-
180948078/#HeRxWPr6A78jhbyD.99
www.ewg.org/guides/cleaners/2234-
CloroxAutomaticToiletBowlCleanerBleachBlueRainClean
www.youtube.com/watch?v=Se12y9hSOM0
www.foreffectivegov.org/chemical-hazards-your-backyard
www.planetnatural.com/lawn-chemicals/
saferchemicals.org/documents/backyard-bbq/
frogsaregreen.org/chemical-pollution-in-your-backyard-researching-
the-effects-of-endocrine-disruptors-in-suburbia/
www.home-air-purifier-expert.com/garage-household-chemicals.html
www.myhealthyhome.com/wp-
content/uploads/2011/02/GARAGE_WHITEPAPER_MASTER.pdf
www.groundwork.org.za/factsheets/toxictour/garage.pdf
my.clevelandclinic.org/health/healthy_living/hic_Steps_to_Staying_We
ll/hic_Household_Chemicals_Chart_Whats_in_my_House
healthylivinghowto.com/1/post/2013/04/healthy-body-7-toxic-
reasons-to-ditch-dryer-sheets.html
www.naturalnews.com/002693_personal_care_products_dryer_sheetl
About 562,000 results (0.52 seconds)
www.healthy-holistic-living.com/72-uses-simple-household-products-
save-money-avoid-toxins.html
eartheasy.com/live_nontoxic_solutions.htm
www.worldwatch.org/system/files/GoodStuffGuide_0.pdf

www.chagrinfallspetclinic.com/2010/07/22/pet-cancer-rates-surging/
www.google.com/#q=cancer+rate+increase+chart
www.wsws.org/en/articles/2003/04/canc-a26.html
articles.mercola.com/sites/articles/archive/2013/06/09/monsanto-
roundup-herbicide.aspx
www.planetnatural.com/lawn-chemicals/ fertilizer
www.globalhealingcenter.com/natural-health/health-dangers-of-dane/
www.epa.gov/indoor-air-quality-iaq/volatile-organic-compounds-
impact-indoor-air-quality
The EPA tested fragrances for chemicals in 1991 and found a list of the
following toxic perfume chemical ingredients: acetone, benzaldehyde,
benzyl acetate, benzyl alcohol, camphor, ethanol, ethyl acetate,
limonene, linalool and methylene chloride – usually in some , 2015
Deadly Scent: Toxic Perfume Chemicals - Mamavation
mamavation.com/2015/03/toxic-perfume-chemicals.html
Does Your Perfume Include Toxic Chemicals? - Mercola
articles.mercola.com/sites/articles/archive/2013/11/27/toxic-perfume-
chem
Nov 27, 2013 - Hidden behind some perfume's pleasant scents are toxic
chemicals linked to hormone disruption, reproductive problems cancer.
Is Your Health Being Destroyed by Other People's Toxic Fragrances?
healthimpactnews.com/.../secondhand-fragrance-contamination-a-
Jun 9, 2014 - Some people love the smell of chemical fragrances, but
30.5% of the ... Heavenly Scents or Toxic Fumes – Are your Fragrances
Healing or ...
Toxic Perfume Chemicals Linked to Cancer, Sperm Damage ...
www.rodalesorganiclife.com/.../toxic-perfume-chemicals-linked-cancer
Perfume ingredients may smell good to some people (while giving
headaches to anyone sensitive to the fumes), but a 2010 study
suggests popular brands
Deadly Scent: Toxic Perfume Chemicals - Mamavation
mamavation.com/2015/03/toxic-perfume-chemicals.html
Mar 18, 2015 - The EPA tested fragrances for chemicals in 1991 and
found a list of the following toxic perfume chemical ingredients:
acetone, benzaldehyde, benzyl acetate, benzyl alcohol, camphor,
ethanol, ethyl acetate, limonene, linalool and methylene chloride –
usually in some combination.
Why Go Fragrance Free? - Invisible Disabilities Association - IDA

invisibledisabilities.org › IDA Books and Pamphlets › Chemical Sensitivities

Then again, most of us do not realize that these fragrances often contain various chemicals that many consider toxic. After all, "Scented FRAGRANCE || Skin Deep® Cosmetics Database | EWG https://www.ewg.org/skindeep/.../FRAGRANCE/ Environmental Working Group

Wildlife and environmental toxicity, EU Ecolabel ... Detergents Ingredients Database ... Fragrance chemicals in domestic and occupational products.

Good Stuff PDF call to action on a Go Green movement. You Asked: Is Perfume Bad for Me? | TIME time.com/3703948/is-perfume-safe/

Feb 11, 2015 - "Look at your perfume bottle and read the ingredients," she suggests. ... Potions that claim to clear your body of toxins might The Danger of Toxic Consumer Products, Fragrances - Huffington Post www.huffingtonpost.com/...s.../toxic-chemicals_b_625648.html graphic – dog in hazmat suite https://koppersgainesville.com/ The Huffington Post

Jul 7, 2010 - Perfumes and fragrances are the single largest category of cosmetic and ... Exposure to toxic ingredients in cosmetics personal Scent of Danger: Are There Toxic Ingredients in Perfumes and ... www.scientificamerican.com/article/toxic-perfumes-and-colognes/ Scientific American

Sep 29, 2012 - To protect trade secrets, makers are allowed to withhold fragrance ingredients, so consumers can't rely on labels to know what h Chemicals and Toxic ingredients in perfumes. Synthetic Free perfume ... www.pourlemondeparfums.com/naturalvssynthetic.html

95% of the chemicals in most commercial fragrances are synthetic compounds derived from petroleum and natural gas, known as petrochemicals. On average ..

People also ask

Is Cologne poison?

Cologne Poisoning. Cologne is a scented liquid made from alcohol and essential oils. Cologne poisoning occurs when someone accidentally or intentionally swallows cologne. This is for information only and not for use in the treatment or management of an actual poison exposure. Cologne Poisoning - The New York Times www.nytimes.com/health/guides/poison/colognes/overview.html

Search for: Is Cologne poison?

What does perfume have in it?

Instead of building a perfume from "ground up", many modern perfumes and colognes are made using fragrance bases or simply bases. Each base is essentially modular perfume that is blended from essential oils and aromatic chemicals, and formulated with a simple concept such as "fresh cut grass" or "juicy sour apple".

Perfume - Wikipedia, the free encyclopedia
en.wikipedia.org/wiki/Perfume

Search for: What does perfume have in it?

What is a synthetic fragrance?

A 1986 report by the National Academy of Sciences reports that 95 percent of the chemicals used in synthetic fragrances are derived from petroleum and include benzene derivatives, aldehydes and many other known toxins and synthesizers capable of causing cancer, birth defects, central nervous system disorders and ...

Essential Oils vs Synthetic Fragrance - Way Out Wax
www.wayoutwax.com/store/pc/viewcontent.asp?idpage=9

Search for: What is a synthetic fragrance?

What is a natural fragrance?

Natural fragrances are essential oils and isolates derived from botanical ingredients that are harvested from the earth such as: flowers, fruits, sap, seeds or skin of the plant, as well as the bark, leaves, roots, resins or wood of certain trees and not from a lab (synthetic).

Natural Perfume vs. Synthetic Perfume - Pour le Monde
www.pourlemondeparfums.com/naturalvssynthetic.html

Search for: What is a natural fragrance?

Searches related to toxic fragrance chemicals

perfume toxic effects

fragrance ingredients toxic

perfume toxicity data

is perfume toxic if swallowed

non-toxic perfumes

perfume toxicity rating

perfume chemicals crossword

safe perfumes

Faircompanies.com
www.washingtonpost.com/national/health-science/study-perc-remains-in-dry-cleaned-clothes/2011/09/01/gIQAbiPsxJ_story.html

www.ewg.org/research/bisphenol
www.ewg.org/news/testimony-official-correspondence/testing-pharmaceuticals-and-personal-care-products-new-york
www.ewg.org/research/flame-retardants-2014/health-dangers
www.ewg.org/news/testimony-official-correspondence/study-almost-half-all-'natural'-personal-care-products
www.ewg.org/research/dog-food-comparison-shows-high-fluoride-
www.ewg.org/successes/2008/breaking-new-ground-toxins-pets
www.dogsnaturallymagazine.com/prescription-pet-foods-found-to-contain-cancer-causing-toxins/
www.dogfoodadvisor.com/red-flag-ingredients/dog-food-
www.petsafe.net/learn/pet-food-the-good-the-bad-and-the-healthy
www.hindawi.com/journals/bmri/2015/234098/
Raising Awareness about Electromagnetic Pollution Marcola.com
http://electromagnetichealth.org
Marcola.com   Are you slowly killing your family
www.scientificamerican.com/article/greener-laundry/
healthypets.mercola.com/sites/healthypets/archive/2010/03/31/dangers-of-flea-and-tick-problems.aspx
Scientist with protective yellow hazmat suit – Shutterstock
Copyright: Lukas Gojda
healthypets.mercola.com/sites/healthypets/archive/2009/09/17/how-cigarettes-and-smoking-impact-your-pets-health.aspx
www.prevention.com/health/healthy-living/electromagnetic-fields-and-your-health
essentialthree.com/blog/?p=595
www.wikihow.com/Dispose-of-Hazardous-Waste
recyclenation.com/2011/04/effective-ways-combat-vocs-recycle-living-room
essentialhealth.com/2012/12/cleaning-your-car-with-essential-oils/
Graphic   animals and world Maria Bell, COLLC0034 clipartof.com
Graphic – polluted world BNP Design Studio, COLLC0148 clipartof.com
Graphic – camel by Cory Thoman, COLLC0121 – clipartof.com
Graphic – Sustainability http://www.zdnet.com/article/a-new-sustainability-resource-the-paper-life-cycle-website/
Graphic – brick house, on a white background by BNP Design Studio, COLLC0148
Graphic- boy and dog running through a neighborhood park by colematt, COLLC0179